Prologue

The dance began suddenly, with a jerk. A spasm, really. A surge of electrical impulse, forcing one thing to jostle into the next, surprising it with power, unsympathetic at first but then soothing through time. Settling into the inevitable. Change. A delta of difference. The way that impulse predicted movement : : predicted feeling : : engendered change : : became dance.

The dance began with a jerk. A wrenching from one state to another; a push and a pull at the same time. This and that, not this or that. Both|and. Movement.

Shaping the change became the province of the dancer. The best dancers manipulated energy to generate motion; they managed the jerking impulses to render electrical variation as aesthetic gesture. Crafting time by shaping the impulses of the body. An alchemy of control and release; a willingness to change and care for the differences in posture, stance, gesture, rhythm. Always rhythm.

Succumbing to the rhythm, enlarging the meter, pounding and denying the beat, resisting its insistence, inhabiting its assumptive logic. Riding it, being with it, chasing it, leading it, following along. The rhythm : : an understanding of form within the jerk.

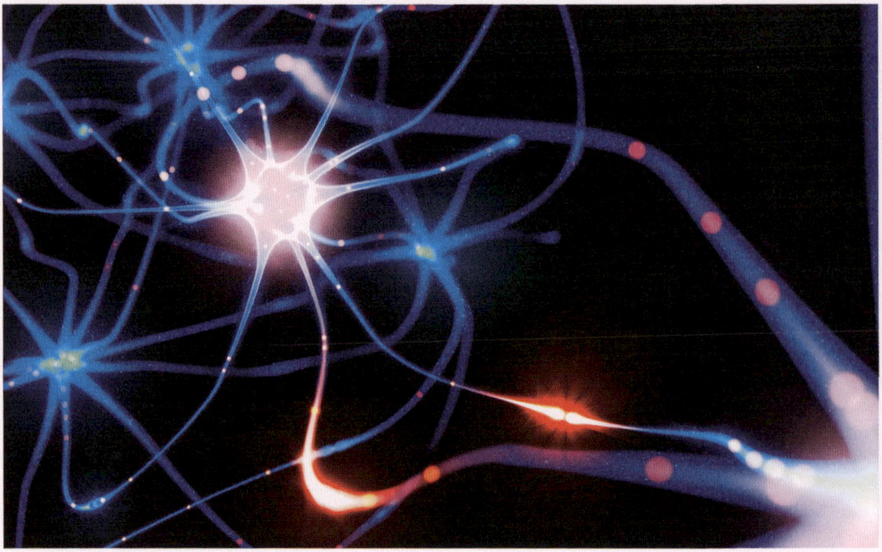

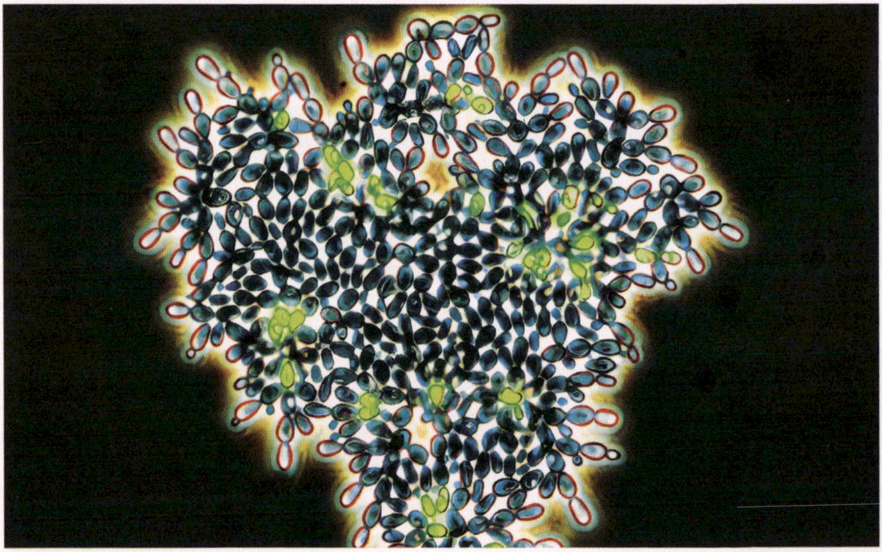

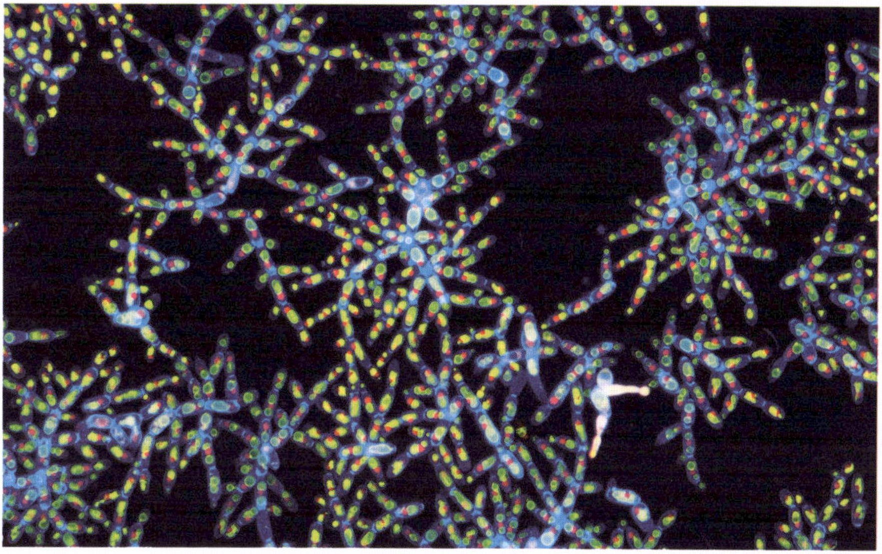

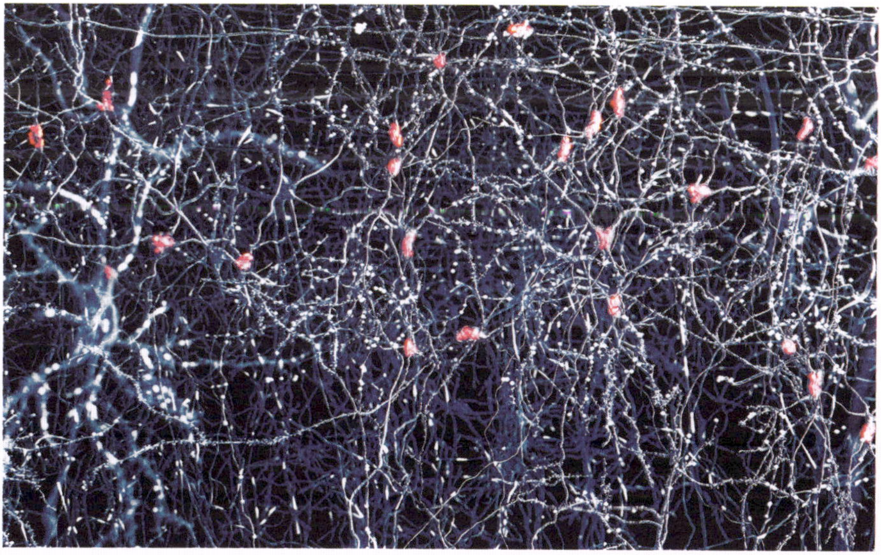

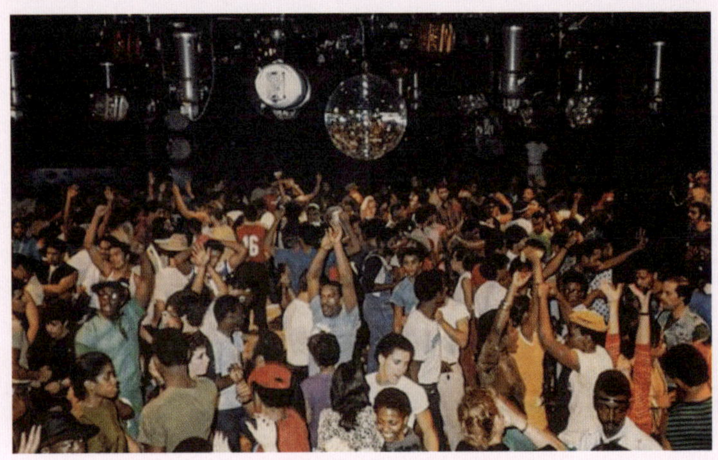

Several Millenia Later...

The electrical impulse that begat dance had been tamed to produce its contents. The flash of the future produced this telling of Black dance history.

...in the Afrofuture, dance instruction is a solitary pursuit...

TeleBrea Roth'astein waved her hand in front of the sensor pad to open the door of the classroom assigned to Arts and Culture 732.5: Black Social Dance. She needed to check the visual-imaging interfaces for her class, scheduled to meet for the first time that evening. TeleBrea was known by a global cohort of students to be a tough but approachable professor of indeterminate age who encouraged her students to understand Black dance as a capacity and strategy more than as a collection of dance forms or set of particular practices. Her interface sessions were smart and sweaty, a combination of discussion, provocation, integrated neural-system participation, and some very old-fashioned dancing. For tonight's session, she expected most of the fifteen hundred enrolled participants from the university and some eighty thousand witnesses, with five live-presence students coming in person to dance in the neural-system-participation classroom.

TeleBrea had been teaching at this private university for only a couple of years. Well, teaching in person, that is. Long ago, she had run a successful neural-distance dance academy of her own. The university had picked up the feed, broadcasting her teaching to its student network as an elective "physical activity." Two years ago, TeleBrea was asked to do on-site sessions. It was highly unusual for someone working in dance—in particular, Black social dance—to be invited to teach on campus. TeleBrea's participation vectors had gone from the twelve hundred she used to have in her broke-down home neuro-pulse network (which operated at a truly slow five million clicks per second) to this brave new hyperfast world of nearly one hundred thousand students

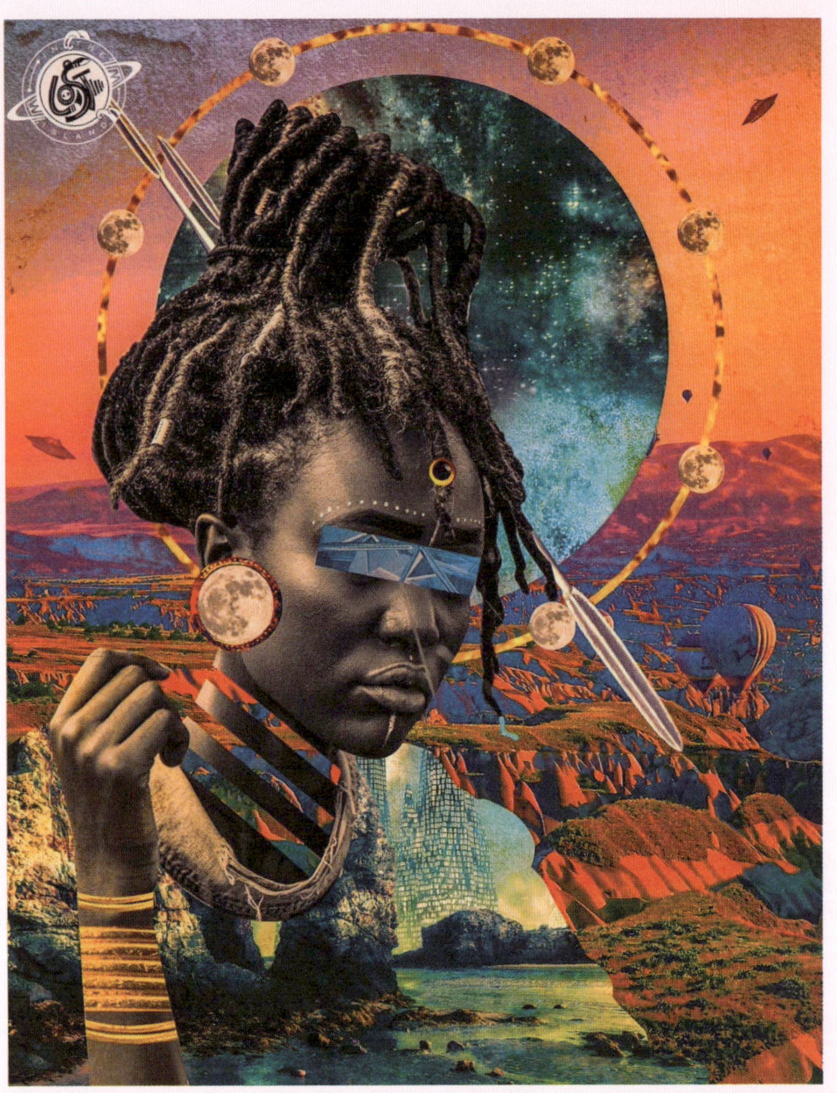

at a time plugged into a full neural interface (two billion responses per second). She liked working in these advanced, freshly outfitted facilities, where, with a tap of her temple processor, she could summon an IT-support team ready to troubleshoot any communication that went awry.

...in the future, dance classes are taught by way of distance neural interfaces as often as not...

Honestly, though, TeleBrea didn't have much experience working with live students in the classroom. TeleBrea's home-teaching sessions had always been conducted without any students in proximity.
The distance neuro-pulse students had tended to be awkwardly detached as they tried to perform the movements she demonstrated, even as their pulse devices guided their gestures via quick nagging electrical charges. Distance dance lessons had become popular when neural implants replaced wearable sensors. As dance teachers generated movement within the very bodies of their students, TeleBrea, like other industrious dance teachers, jumped onto the bandwagon of impulse-driven instruction. The emergent technological interfaces allowed more and more people to take up dancing as creative physical exercise. The plug-and-play method of having a talented dancer literally move you by way of her movement attracted all sorts of students.

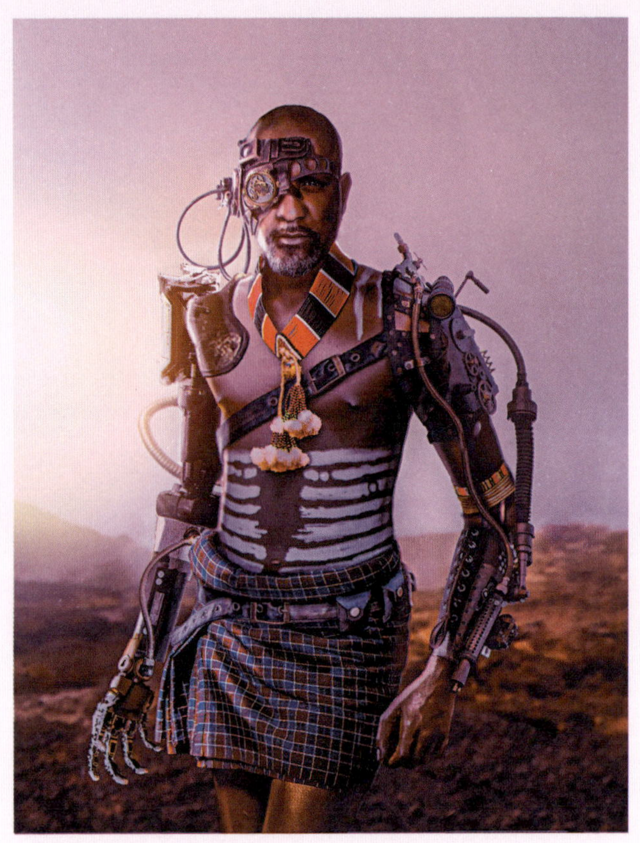

. . . in the Afrofuture, traditional Black social dance is still taught body to body—at home . . .

TeleBrea's specialty was the old-timey Black dances of the twenty-first century. She learned these dances from her father, Zekeil, when she was a little boy. Zekeil came from a dancing family. In fact, TeleBrea's parents had met at a dancing protest in New Detroit. Zekeil and Jadeena, TeleBrea's mother, danced at all the protests they could in the 2070s: at the resistance against Central Congo overdevelopment, at the

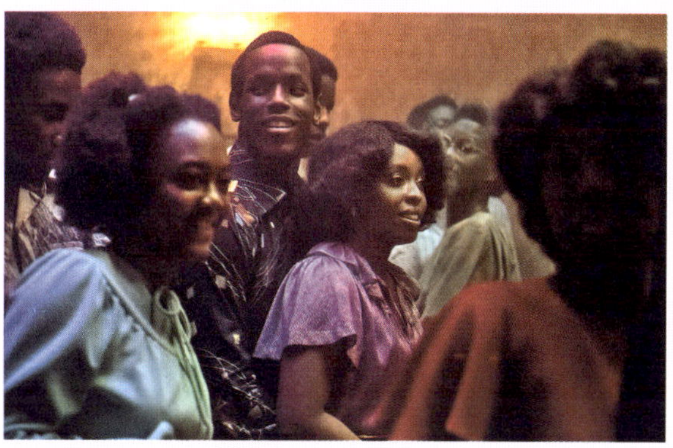

rethinking-repatriation affair of South Florida, at the holistic happiness hoedown staged in Chinese Côte d'Ivoire.

When TeleBrea was born, Zekiel and Jadeena knew that he was no single-gender child, and they did the work to allow him to express the gender-fluid identities that suited him. Intragender children were not all that uncommon at the dawn of the twenty-second century, but the dispersed community didn't make anyone's life easier. Between five and eight years old, TeleBrea preferred to be recognized as a boy, and Zekeil taught him the basics of turn-of-the-last-century b-boying as best he could. Zekeil learned them from the old World War IV internet archives you could still find hooked up to some church communication networks. He taught him the wind-jamming line dances that had been popular in the 2030s, the great power-failure decade, when most Black folk lived with electricity only half the time. And he taught him the man-to-man be-a-man partner dances that had developed in the megajails of the 2060s, those dances that alternated tender-caressing hand-dancing and full-bodied slamdancing, crashing one into the other to the synthesized sounds of the mechanical apocalypse. TeleBrea enjoyed these styles and how his father guided him through the movements the old way by demonstrating, playing together, discussing the metaphor and meaning, and touching hand-shoulder-leg-foot-elbow-hip-forehead.

TeleBrea learned her warrior dances from her grandmother Tesladella Roth'astein, her mama's mama, who had emigrated from Argentina in the 2050s. Tesladella taught TeleBrea the long-time-ago Black Power fertility and power dances: twerking and j-setting. Learning these dances from her grammamere helped TeleBrea understand her feminine and social self as a capacity she had to practice. In the middle of a vogue drop—a movement she always did as part of her twerk sequence—TeleBrea thought of herself as a badass girlboy, ready to kick the ass of racist bs worldwide and across time.

...in the Afrofuture, some dancers claim mixed-gender, mixed-race Blackness...

TeleBrea's social dance classes gained in popularity as he matured as a mixed-gender mediated personality. He began posting his 3-D-visualization dance logs as a teenager, first alternating gender representation week by week and then day by day. She didn't want her gender shifting to be a trick, so she always chose a unified mode each day, sometimes something recognizably male, surreptitiously androgynous, but demonstrably female, other times straight-up fembot glamour-puss. Her glamour-puss persona, while popular, took considerable time to generate, and TeleBrea only worked that mode on rare occasion. TeleBrea's claim to Blackness, though, never wavered.

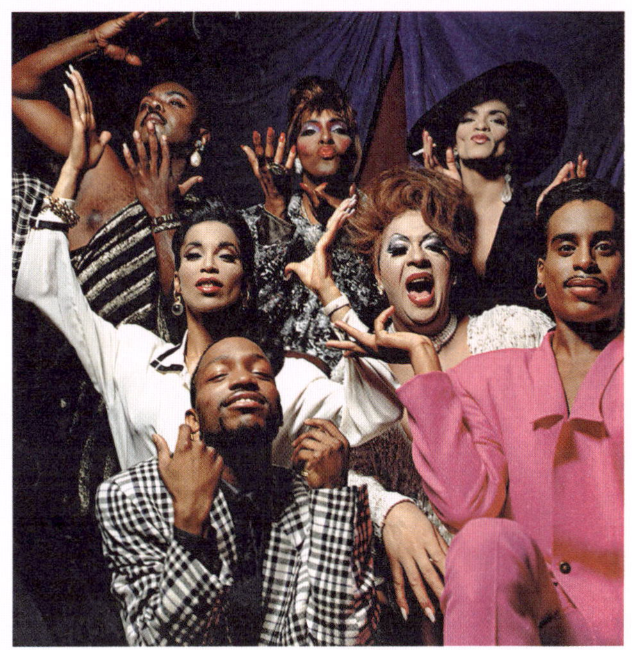

...in the Afrofuture, neural attachments allow students to connect with instructors at the level of muscular impulse...

The five on-site student teaching assistants freaked TeleBrea out. They were young, hungry for movement, agile, and, she thought, not very nice. Of course, they each had excellent technique and could do pretty much anything that came their way. They were all hyperflexible, and a couple of them could dislocate their shoulders on command to perform the old MarsMan styles that blew up in the 2140s. The university assigned these TAs to TeleBrea without her consultation, and they were paid with tuition remission and superfast neural-connection interfaces. The TAs provided an alternative physical narrative for the distance learners; students could alternate between the impulses that TeleBrea emitted and those of any of the TAs. TeleBrea knew her dancing

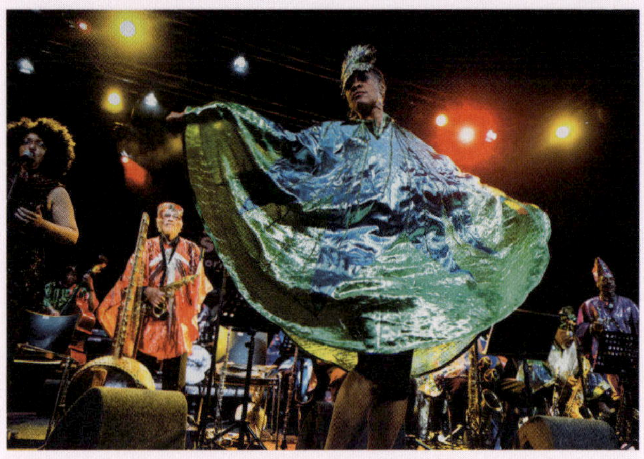

was infinitely more nuanced than that of the TAs, but many of the course enrollees preferred to feel the spikes of energy cast by the younger dancers.

Teaching, TeleBrea relaxed into remembering the dances and engaging their contours. She dipped with subtlety and suppleness, carefully tending to the motions and their implications, narrating the histories as she had been taught them and demonstrating their bounded weightiness, rhythmicity, and affect.

On this particular day, she chose to focus on the oldest dance in her repertoire, a strangely free-floating but rhythmic partner dance from the old days. TeleBrea knew his Black history, and he knew that this was a dance about the prison-industrial complex and the ways that twenty-first-century Black youth would engage in extravagant gang dance battles. The dance called for a sort of weighted-volition down-and-back, down-and-back with the legs, while the arms floated and pushed, the hands gathered into loose fists, and the chest heaved in time to a sound score of dogs barking and old police sirens.

TeleBrea danced, and the TAs looked bored. She knew that they would rather be doing their bumping-time interface dances, the ones that gave full-body stimulation by neural feedback in

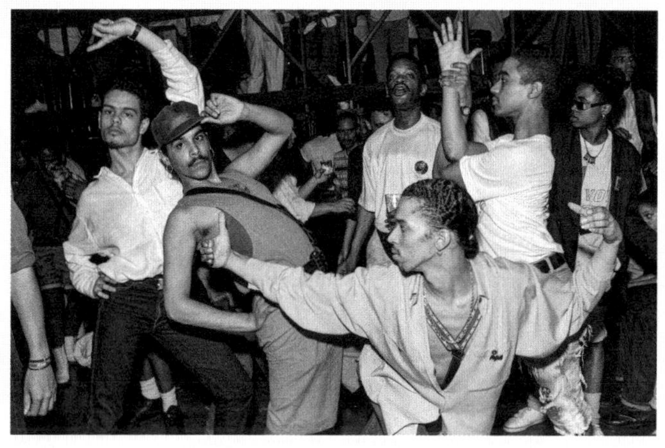

response to the slightest passing erotic thought. Some folks thought of these new styles as just sex dances that interfaced young people did together in groups of eighty to ninety, and that they were nothing more than electronic orgies that had nothing to do with dancing and little to do with Black culture. TeleBrea wasn't sure. Maybe there was something in this group undulation that had emerged in a hookup network between Oakland and South Memphis and that told a story about Black erotic connection? One time, she switched on her feedback paradigm, which allowed her to feel the gestures that her students created, to better understand where the movements worked and, more commonly, where they didn't. Sure enough, while most of her students were trying to capture the gestures she created, others were watching interface news feeds or chatting about music.

TeleBrea did the unusual. She screwed up her face, clenched her fists, deepened her voice, and morphed into a male persona. "Come on now, wake up!" he said. "This is an important dance you need to know to understand Black history! This is an old courtship dance that would be done by partners who wanted to get each other's attention. Jack your legs, heave your chest, make a loose fist, and push up alongside your partner so you can dance in team. Let's go now, this is it. It's time to do... the RUNNING MAN!"

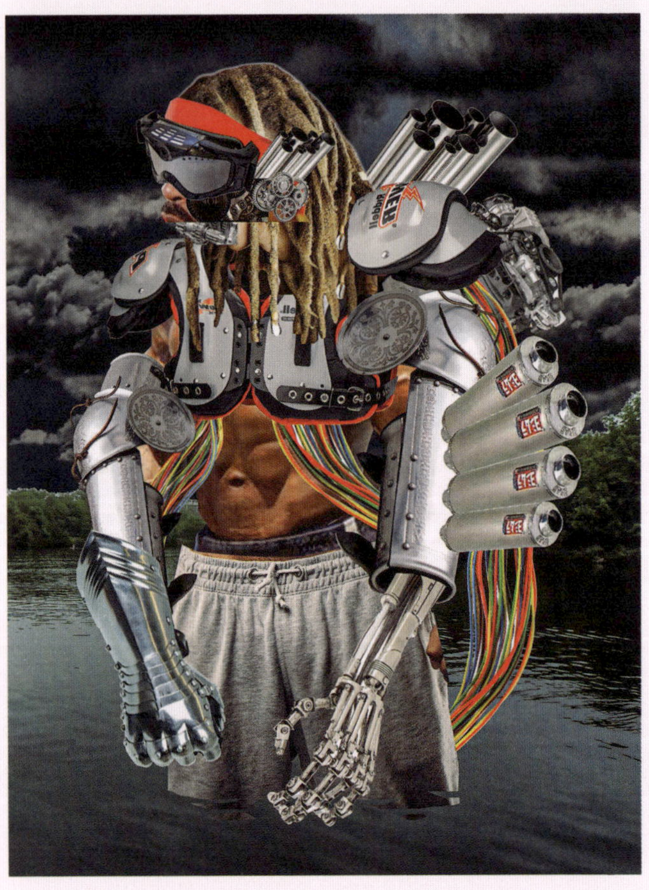

...Later That Time Cycle...

TeleBrea had learned dance history both ways. She had scoured the legal and illegal blockchains that held normative and manufactured renderings of the pasts. The documented accountings of where dance had emerged and where it had been supported. The dancing ceremonies that allowed girls to become young women in Yorubaland; the circle events that allowed communities to celebrate ground, grain, time, wind, ancestors, and corn in the First Nations. She knew about the courts and political regimes that used dance as a weapon in Old-Old Europe, the ways that dance kept people in their place according to ability in those systems.

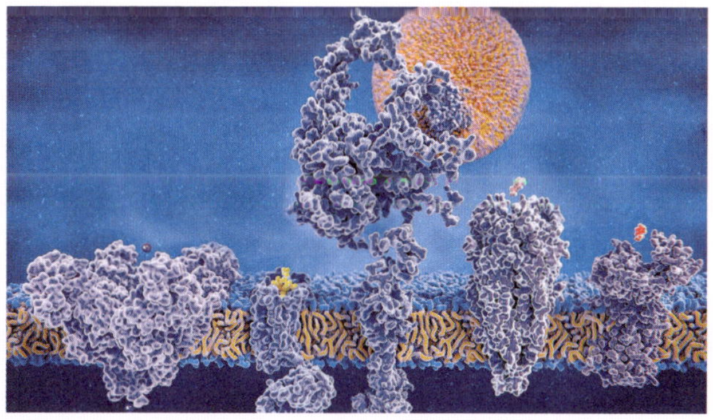

In Old-Old Europe, the blockchains showed, monarchs forced dance onto the ruling classes, judging their faults harshly and barely rewarding achievement. In the more recent Old Europe, tyrants forced dance onto the working masses, demanding military parades and spectacles of movement that revealed monstrous visions of anonymous power. New Europe hadn't been much better, in TeleBrea's view, with its daily protest mosh pits, which always left at least a few thousand souls injured. Dance was a constant throughout all these histories there were to know.

TeleBrea learned dance history the other way too, the more dangerous way. She asked people what they remembered. And she danced with them. She sought out people through the neural-pathway emitters whenever they mentioned dance in a context that signaled something from before the Last Revision. Traveling to visit people wasn't always taken kindly, but the old people TeleBrea sought out didn't seem to mind much. Most of them had avoided the implants that connected billions of others through an electrical interface. The implants allowed the giant global conglomerates to flourish. Corporations had long since replaced nation-states, but some people still understood that place and the rituals of location matter.

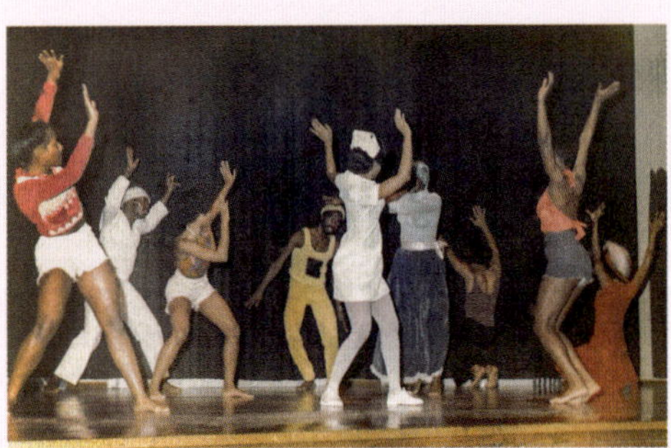

Dancing with others, TeleBrea learned stories of important figures from the distant past who had a lasting impact on how people decided to move together. And that's what dance history had always been, she thought—a decision to move together.

She learned about Bob Johnson of Old Pittsburgh and Rod Rodgers of First New York. She knew that they had made dances during the Black Arts Movement of the 1960s and 1970s and that they made dances that were not about themselves but about things they imagined. That sort of dancing was only popular for one hundred fifty years or so. After the First Climate Collapse, people really only danced about themselves.

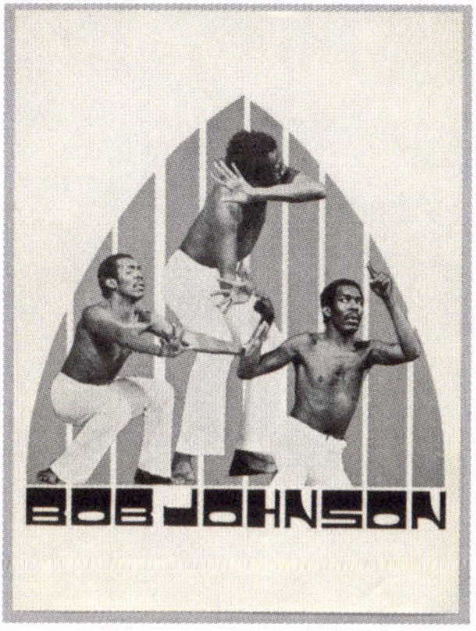

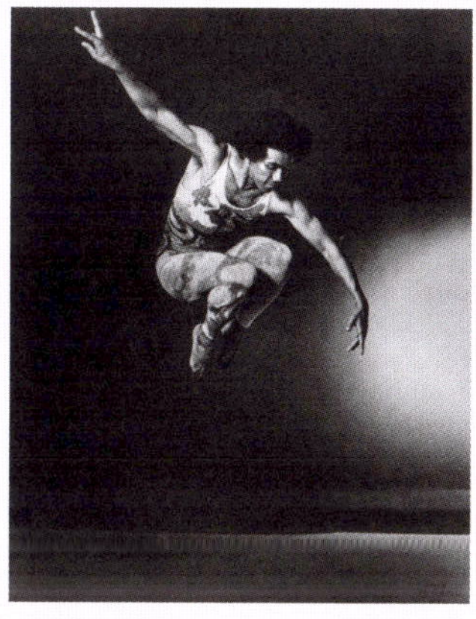

She learned about Lester Horton, who had a cabaret dance theater in Original Los Angeles, and who mixed races and sexualities among his colleagues. Horton mattered because he brought together the crowd that surrounded him. Most people surrounded themselves with people who were just like themselves in terms of size, skin, hair, age, and general attitude. Horton had done something else again, bringing together people who had no real need to meet except that he made space for this to happen.

She learned about Mary Bruce, who ran a dance studio in Harlem and taught hundreds of Black children and young adults for a half century. Bruce created a social possibility by sharing dance and introducing people to experiences they had dreamed about, like performing at Carnegie Hall.

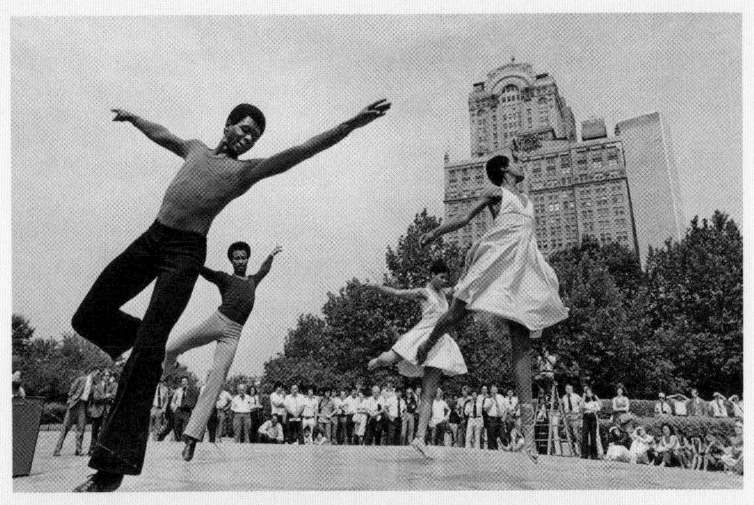

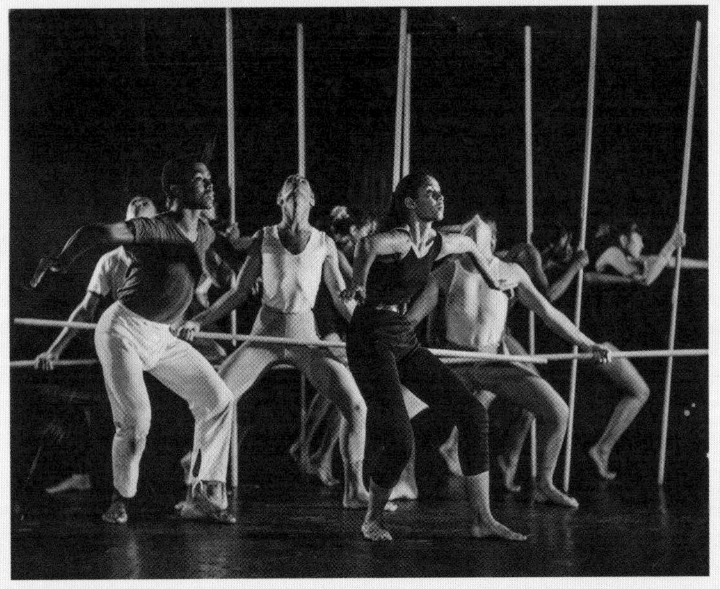

She learned about Ada Overton Walker (sometimes called Aida), who choreographed productions on Broadway in the 1900s. Once called "the best Negro comedienne today," Walker, who worked as a celebrity dance artist and was a well-known tastemaker, was an activist and advocate for Black femme presence. Walker illusioned gender well.

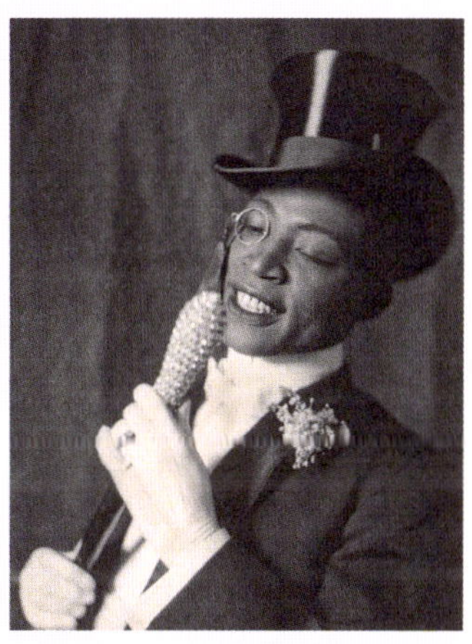

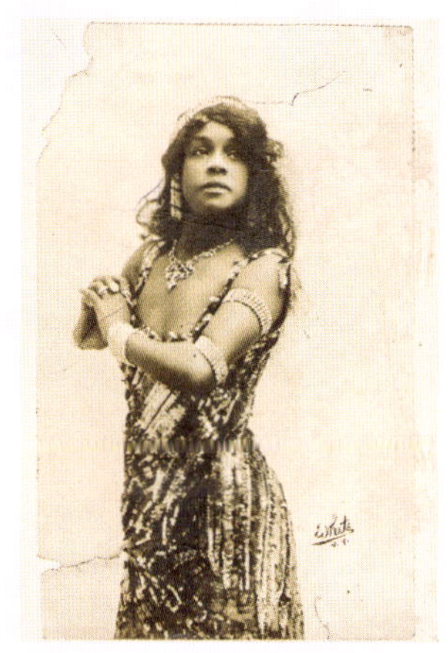

She learned about the most famous near-forgotten artists, with names like Alvin Ailey, Katherine Dunham, and Pearl Primus, who launched a global commitment to Black theatrical dance in the awkward days of the twentieth century.

Learning, TeleBrea felt super femme. Like dance itself, which was usually gendered female, TeleBrea took the telling of dance history as an essentially feminist practice, a way to "spend time" in reflection and communion without needing to know an outcome. A place to experiment and feel. A place to wander in spirit.

The oldest dance that mattered to Black people in the First United States was a spirit form that intrigued TeleBrea to no end. A dance that evolved from circles within circles, traveling against the clock, rewinding time with shouts and cries, screams and songs, improvisations and elaborations of pain and triumph. A dance that involved men, women, children, and all the permutations that produce a people in motion and feeling the spirit: the ring shout. If only, TeleBrea thought, the students could come to experience something of the complete deliverance offered by that most ancient of forms.

No matter now, though. Dance history is a moving target without end. What came before the ring shout were the slave ships; and before that, the tribal disagreements and ritual disputes; and before that, the confusions of change through time that exceeded what anyone could ever really know, let alone understand. Living in dance, TeleBrea learned the essential lesson: dance histories are chronicles of people moving beyond what they think they know.

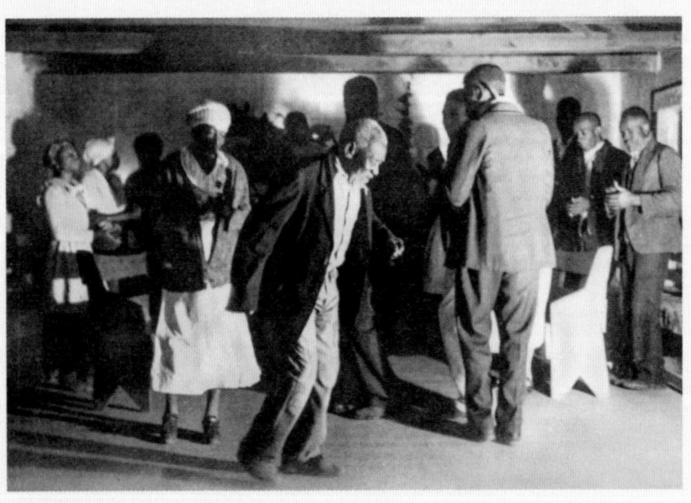

Afterword

TeleBrea eventually stopped teaching and capitulated to a full-consciousness dissolve into the data network. It wasn't an easy decision to join the streaming hordes of once-living beings, but electrical connections promised an even greater capacity to stretch across time and space. For the gender-shifting populace, data dissolves allowed for a simultaneity that suited an eagerness to be more than one or two. Dancers often performed the dissolve and claimed to enjoy playing among the rolling tides of power that embraced the dissolved and allowed them to surge, congregate, survey, and disperse in rhythms of exploration.

Eventually, TeleBrea disassembled. In time, the dissolved stopped being recognizable. They joined the electrical current as pure motivation, as an impulse, a jolt. The dispersal took a while, though. In a few hundred cycles, there might be none to remember the coherent resolve that had been the dance expert TeleBrea.

Except for one thing. A glitch in the system. A portion of TeleBrea's dance history remained intact in the blockchain; one idea following the next in a minor assembly. No one could know how it happened. A fragment of consciousness, telling a story of dance, survived the inevitable dispersal. This is what it said:

I wanted to dance with others and to share the smell of our excitement, to place a hand on the small of a back and smile as we stepped this way, then that, together. I wanted to engage in the most human of activities, to shape time by playing with rhythm. I wanted to love, and care, and wonder in our moving, and I wanted to show others what I thought I could do and who I wanted to be, by dancing. I wanted that revelation for them. I wanted that for us. I wanted to teach them the dance that my studies made me care for the most: the dance of the group as a bulbous, differentiated assembly, each doing as they will with all of us dancing together. Right and right and right and right. Left and left and left and left. Back two three four. Step touch, step back, step turn. Repeat and repeat and repeat until we are all happy beyond life, full of potential, full of relation, full of emotion. We slide, people, we Electric Slide. Right and right and right and right. Left and left and left and left. Back two three four. Step touch, step back, step turn. Slide, people, slide. rightandrightandright andright. leftandleftandleftandleft. backtwo threefour. steptouchstepbackstepturn. SLIDE! rghtrghtrghtrght. lftlftlftlftlfft. bk234. sttchstbksttn. SLIDE. rnrnrnr. lnlnlnl. b234. stsbst. SLIDE. rnrnrnr. lnlnlnl. b234. stsbst. SLIDE. rnrnrnr. lnlnlnl. b234. stsbst. SLIDE. rrrr. llll. b2-4. stsbst. SLIDE.

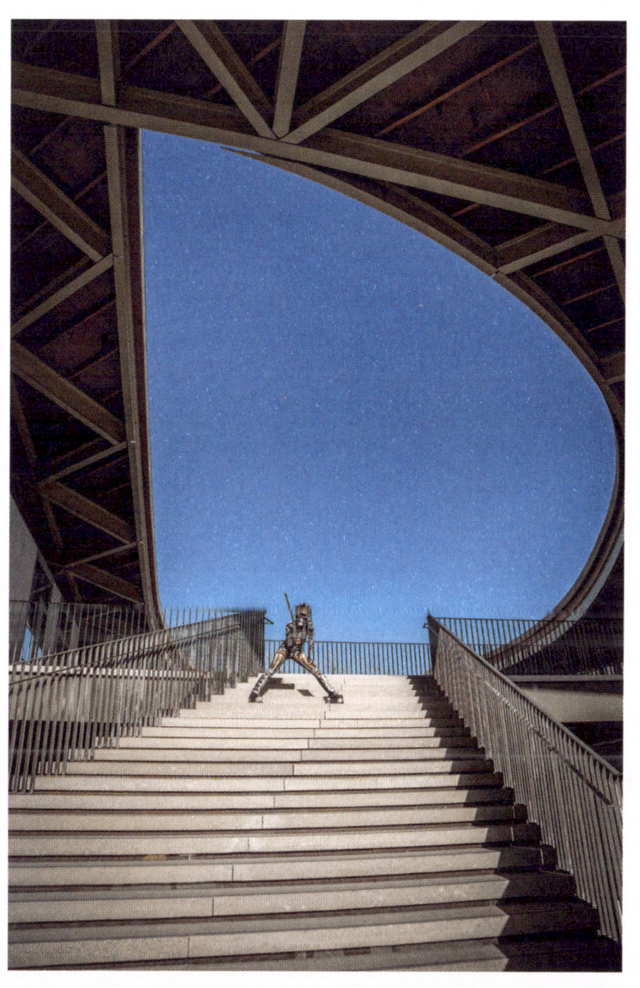

IMAGES

Page 2 (top): Nerve cells and electrical pulses. Image: KTSDESIGN/ Science Photo Library via Getty Images
Page 2 (bottom): Green cells undergoing cell death, a cellular division of labor fostering new life. Image: Will Ratcliff and Mike Travisano, courtesy National Science Foundation
Page 3 (top): Unicellular yeast evolving into multicellular "snowflake yeast" collectives. Image: Georgia Institute of Technology, Atlanta
Page 3 (bottom): Neuron network in the human brain. Image: selvanegra/iStock
Page 4: The Paradise Garage, New York, 1981
Page 6: © Kaylan Michel
Page 8: Serengeti cyborg, by Solen Feyissa, https://www.flickr.com/photos /solen-feyissa/50040111491
Page 9: Still of Michael Ward and Amarah-Jae St. Aubyn in "Lovers Rock," episode two of *Small Axe*, dir. Steve McQueen, 2020. Courtesy Steve McQueen
Page 11: Film still from *Paris Is Burning*, 1990, dir. Jennie Livingston © Off White Productions/ Courtesy Everett Collection
Page 12: Sun Ra Centennial Dream Arkestra, performing at North Sea Jazz Festival, Rotterdam, Netherlands, July 12, 2014. Photo by Dimitri Hakke/Redferns via Getty Images
Page 13: Voguers Luis, Danny, Jose, and David-Ian of House of Xtravaganza, New York, May 1989. Photo © Chantal Regnault
Page 14: © Stacey A. Robinson
Page 15: Structure variety of membrane proteins. Image: Juan Gaertner/ Shutterstock.com
Page 16, 17 (left): Bob Johnson Papers, 1949–2003, CTC.2014.03, Curtis Theatre Collection, Archives & Special Collections, University of Pittsburgh Library System
Page 17 (right): Rod Rodgers, photo by Jack Mitchell. Courtesy and © Kim Grier-Martinez/ Rod Rodgers Dance Company
Page 18 (top): The Rod Rodgers Dance Company performing in Battery Park, 1975. Photo by Tyrone Dukes, courtesy and © Kim Grier-Martinez/ Rod Rodgers Dance Company
Page 18 (bottom): Lester Horton's *Liberian Suite* (1952), performed by Alvin Ailey City Center Dance Theater, 1975. Photo by Charles van Maanen. Lester Horton Dance Theater Collection, Music Division, Library of Congress
Page 19 (left): Cavendish Morton, *George W. Walker in "In Dahomey,"* 1903. Platinotype print, 6½ × 4¾ inches. National Gallery
Page 19 (right): Aida Overton Walker as Salome, c. 1911. Photo by White Studio, © Billy Rose Theatre Division, The New York Public Library for the Performing Arts
Page 20: Gullah Geechee ring shout, c. 1930. Photo by Maxfield Parrish Jr. Courtesy of Lorenzo Dow Turner Papers, Anacostia Community Museum Archives, Smithsonian Institution
Page 23: ZiggZaggerZ the Bastard (cosplay), 2019. Photo by tobias c. van Veen.

In the Beginning, Everyone Danced

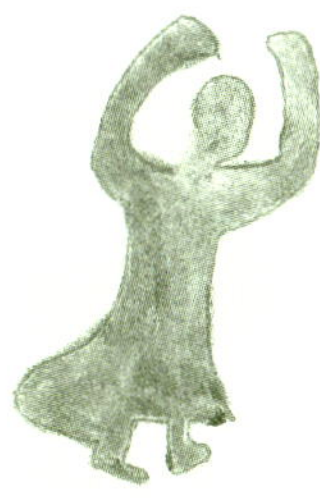

This is a drawing I made of a dance from 6000 BCE

In the beginning, everyone danced. People danced for rain, for fertility, for celebration. They danced for a good harvest and success in battle. They danced to meet, to marry, to bind, and to bury; they danced for their well-being, and they danced to bring their communities together for safety and harmony. Thousands of years ago, everyone danced. And everything that was vitally important in life had a dance associated with it. Life was marked by and depended on dancing. These dances were acts of living. Hope, fear, pleasure, survival—this was the beginning of dance. Dance was fundamental. Dance mattered.

Who were the first dancers? Birds, insects, fish; all animals have choreographic actions that function aesthetically and biologically. Dance is of nature; dance is natural.

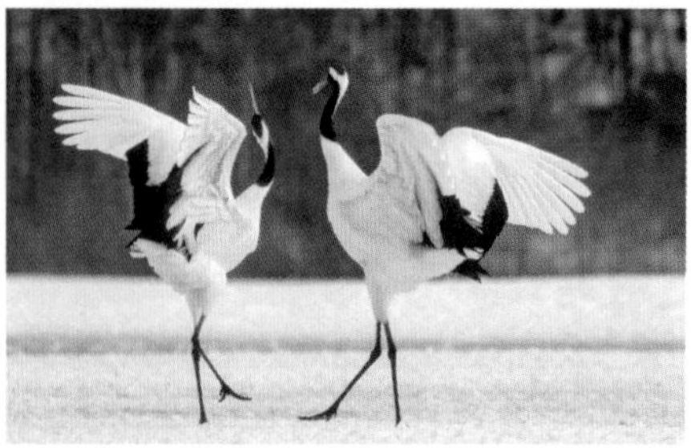

This is a duet.

Symbolic and asymbolic dance forms, repeated, learned, and passed down, addressed fundamental matters of fertility, food, and safety. The passing down of these dances—teaching and learning dance—was central to growing up. The successful hunt or harvest could be attained through dancing—*if* the dancing was done fully and well. And the separation between watching dance and *doing* dance was nonexistent. Everyone danced.

Fast-forward thousands of years to ancient Greece

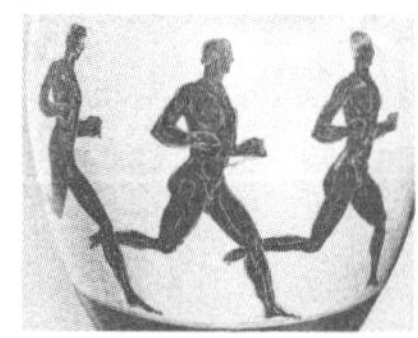

Socrates Danced. Plato Danced. Everyone Danced.

The ancient Greeks had elaborate systems of dance. They divided their dances into two categories: peace dance and war dance.

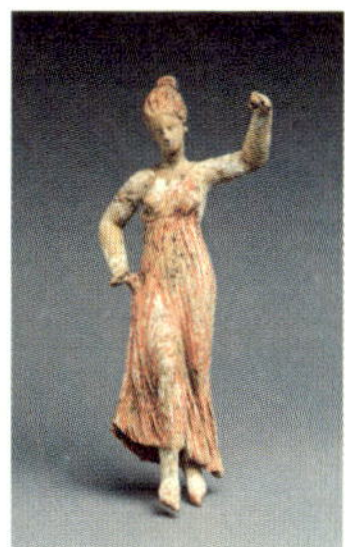

This is a peace dance.

Dance was part of military training. Large-scale unison movement was intended not only to bind and empower a group from within but also to intimidate, to get bigger.

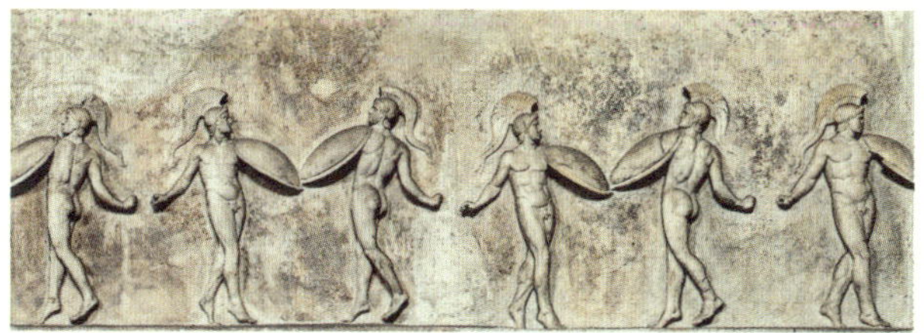

This is a war dance.

More than two hundred dances are named in the texts of ancient Greece, and these dances were taught in school.

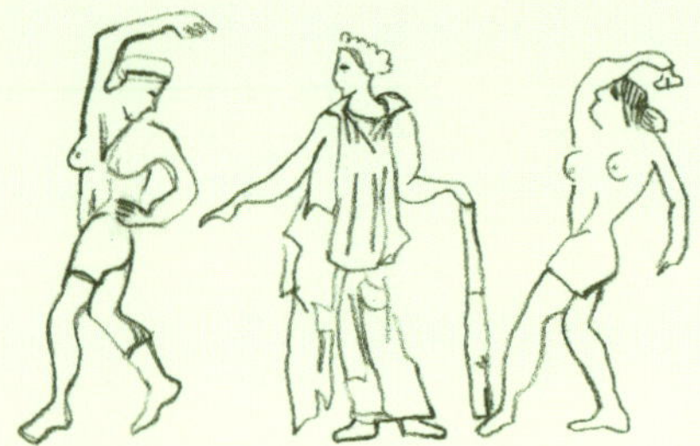

Dance class has been going on for a very long time.

The Greeks illustrated their dances on pots.

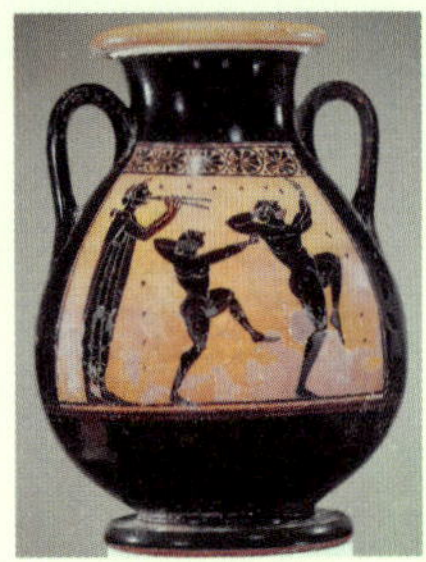

Pots were the social media of ancient Greece.

Soldiers danced.
Philosophers danced.
Everyone danced.

Fast-forward
hundreds
of years

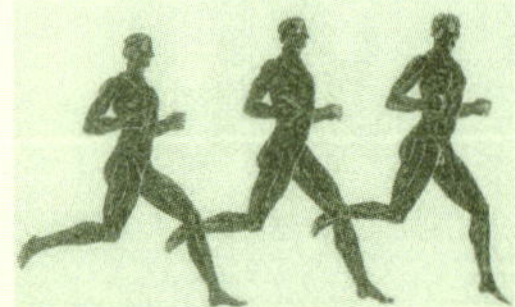

Jesus Danced

Like everyone, Jesus danced. This aspect of Jesus's life has been essentially erased from the New Testament. But Jesus did dance, and his dancing and what he said about the power of dance are reported in the once-censored Gnostic Gospels. It could be that writings about dancing were left out of the official Christian documents because dance might be seen as female, chaotic, sublime, and powerful—all things that might serve the greater good but not the formation of unilateral patriarchy.

Here, Jesus describes the power and insight that dancing gives you:

> *Thou that dancest, perceive what I do....*
> *Ye who dance* not *know* not *what we are knowing....*
> *If you respond to my dance, see yourself in me*
> *as I speak, and if you have seen what I do, keep silent*
> *about my mysteries. You who dance, understand*
> *what I do for yours is this human passion I am about*
> *to suffer.... Now answer thou unto my dancing...*
> *and seeing what I do, keep silence about my mysteries.*
> (Acts of John, 96–97)

Here is a recounting of a circle dance that occurred as a final ritual just before Jesus was crucified:

> *He bade us therefore make as it were a ring,*
> *holding one another's hands, and himself*
> *standing in the midst.... Thus, having danced*
> *with us the Lord went forth.* (Acts of John, 94–97)

Fast-forward
a thousand
years

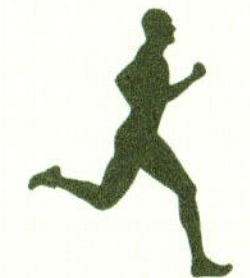

Hold Hands and Hop

In medieval Europe, dance was largely distilled to simple circles and lines, stepping, sliding, ducking, and hopping to rhythms. Variations of these directives abound from culture to culture.

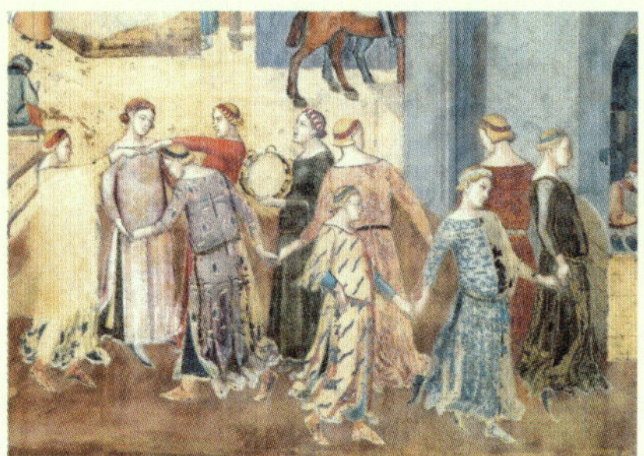

This is a variation of a circle dance in the Middle Ages.

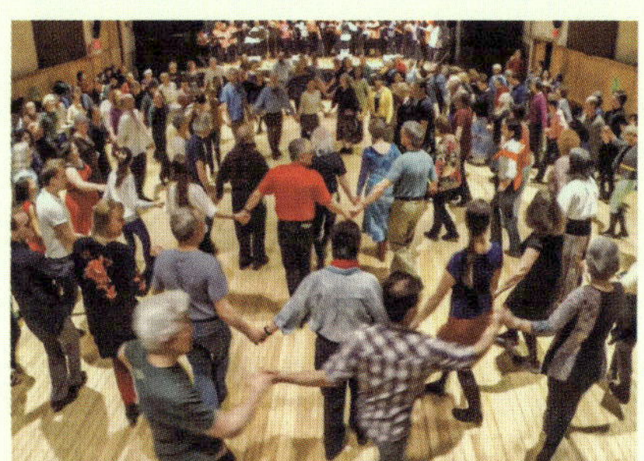

We still do this.

Q: Why, for thousands of years, have people worn flowers in their hair, held hands, and hopped in a circle like these Morris dancers in Trafalgar Square?

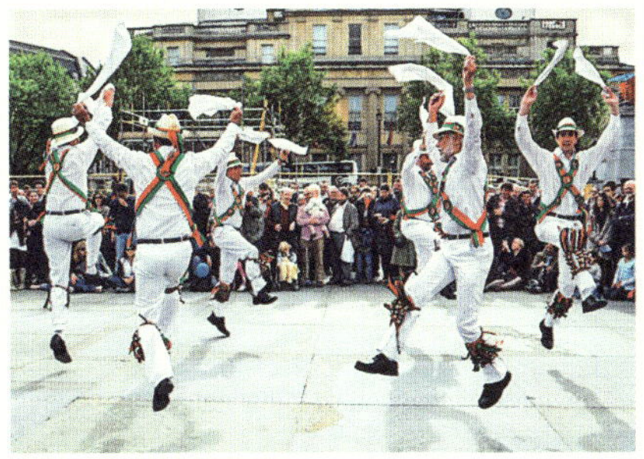

The answer is both physical and metaphysical.

Skip ahead

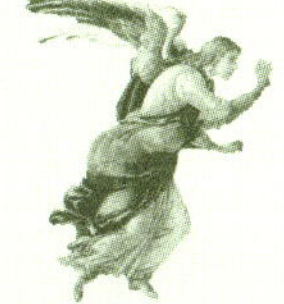

The Room in the Renaissance

For thousands of years, everyone danced,

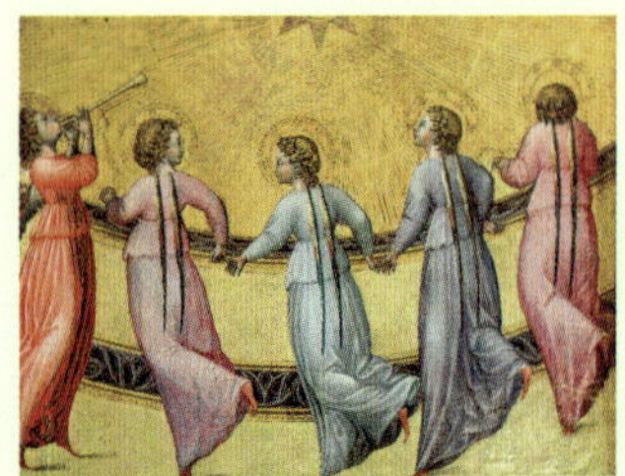

including angels.

Then, one day, dance went indoors, and people danced in rooms. And these rooms were divided into two parts. On one side of the room, people stopped dancing and sat down. And on the opposite side of the room, the other people danced for them. In this radical shift in dance history, dance acquired not only a stage and an audience but also an economy and a gatekeeper. And with this new spatial configuration, dance became Art, and people became creators of new forms of it.

But what was <u>it</u>?

It was choreography, the aesthetic and intentional organization of the body in space.

Fast-forward to the nineteenth century

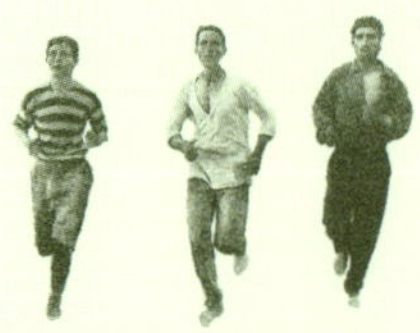

Wings, Wands, and Feathers

In the European nineteenth century, elaborate renderings of magical, moralistic, and angsty narratives, organized into large-scale regal movement, romanticized life's grit. The predominant subject matter was floating, flying fairies, princes, princesses, and magic. Wings, wands, feathers, and flowers, things puffy, pink, and related to dreams were the stuff of this moment.

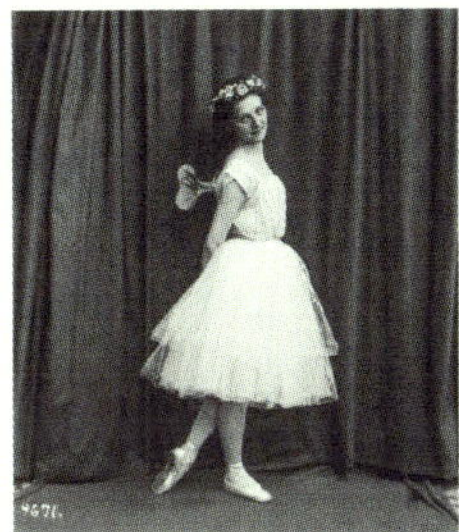

This dancer is pretending to be a fairy.

A new technology developed to express these ideas: the toe shoe. The toe shoe suggests a yearning for departure through lift and antigravity; it makes one feel immortal and not of this fearful Earth.

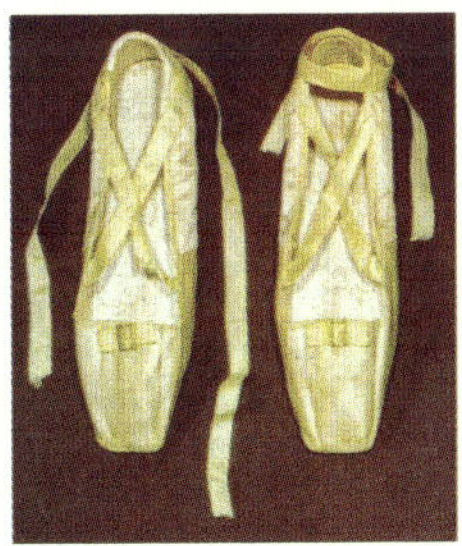

A new technology.

The Sense of Nonsense

In the early twentieth century, European artists witnessed firsthand "sophisticated" cultures descend into shocking barbarity. Artists saw World War I as a war devoid of meaning, characterized by brutal absurdity. The Dadaists brilliantly made this meaninglessness literal; they used the stage to make their own sense out of nonsense. Blurring genres, visual artists choreographed by referring to and simultaneously rejecting ballet technique as a dead, hierarchical relic of the "system" that had failed them. Rationality itself was proven illogical and dangerous in practice, and the Dadaists embraced this paradox by dismantling notions of what was logical and virtuosic in their art. Their work embraced flatness, repetition, and non-narrative sequencing.

Triadisches Ballett (1912) is a ballet by Oskar Schlemmer.

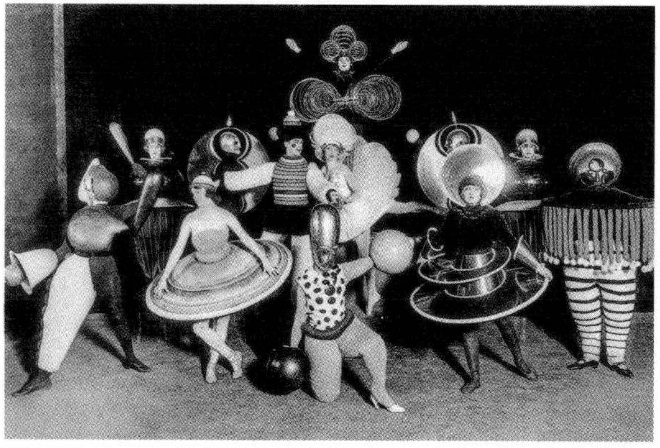

This dance is committed to nonmeaning.

Twentieth-Century America: The Ground, the Gaze

In America, however, Freud permeated the dancers' emotions. So did Jung's idea of the archetypal self. In response, dance makers rejected the heavenly aspirations of the nineteenth century in favor of looking deep within the human; they took off their shoes to connect to the Earth. This was the period of the primal, the elemental, the ground. The emotionality of the human back became central to dance vocabulary. The limbs responded to the torso rather than the torso responding to the limbs.

Lamentations (1930) is a modern dance by Martha Graham.

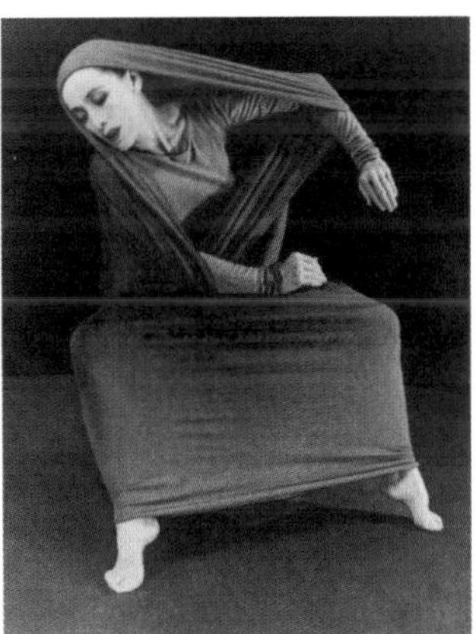

This dance is about internal struggle.

Trees

Imagine two distinct forests in the family trees of dance, one devoted to nostalgia and the other to expressing the present as it truly is.

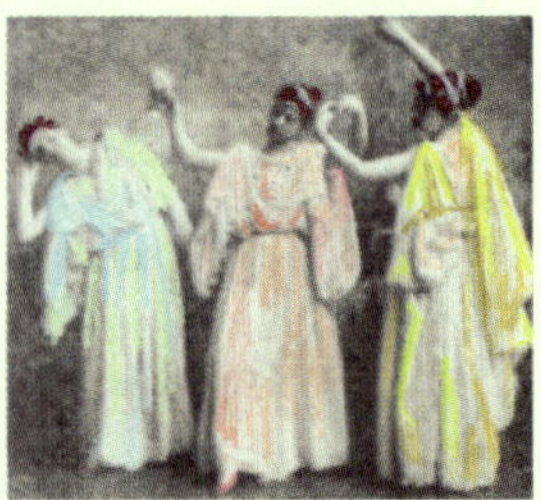

This is a dance from the family tree devoted to looking back.

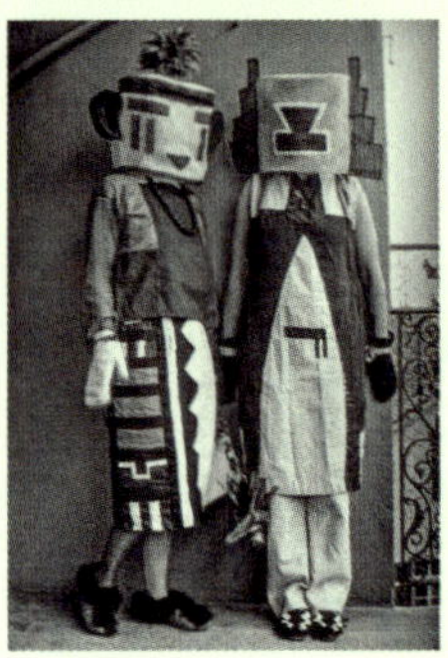

Here Sophie Taeuber-Arp references ancient Hopi patterns, as she upends Western ideas of costuming—an ancient practice in itself.

Note: *A branch structure is a natural structure that occurs in nature. The lungs, the veins in your hand, the act of thinking, a conversation, and a tree all have branching structures. And this structure also occurs in dance history. Dance movements and makers could be loosely grouped into family trees.*

But it doesn't work to hold onto this tree metaphor; it's overly organized. Some artists don't fit neatly into any family tree. Before modernism, Gertrude Stein invented postmodernism. Though not a dance maker, Stein's extreme experiments in upending grammar and syntax have left a mark on every postmodern dance I have ever made or watched—though this probably means she has left an indelible mark on my mind.

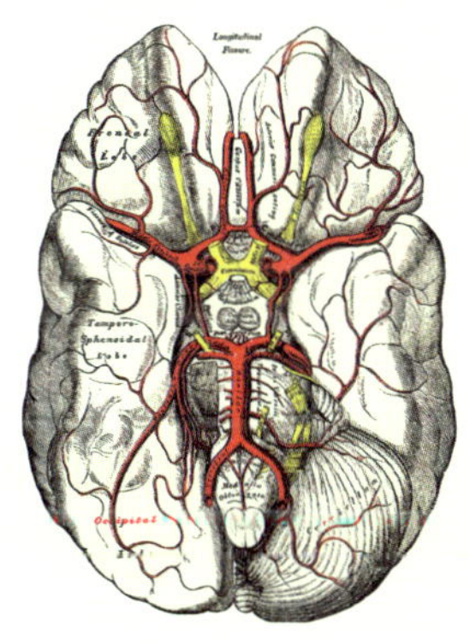

Fast-forward to the second half of the twentieth century

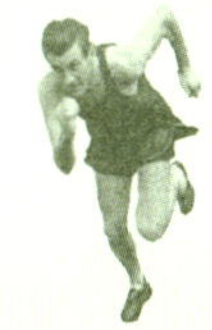

The Ashen Body in Space

On a small island in northern Japan, a new dance form emerged from the rubble of World War II, a form so disciplined, primal, and intense as almost to deny the notion of breath in the body. This dance form is named butoh, or "dance of darkness, dance of death," and it depicts the self as a body surfaced from the ruin of the Earth—naked, smeared with white ashes, in decay, barely alive. After that war, nothing more than this could possibly have occurred—no dynamics, no crescendos, no morality, no fairies, and no psychology. Duration, slowness, and stillness were explored; walking itself became a strange act.

Kazuo Ohno was a founder of butoh. Beautifully unpredictable, he portrayed (over and over again) a great female flamenco artist, La Argentina. Fetal, tottering in heels, hunched back, in a broken glamour, his dance was an oblique nod to the destruction of something great and complicated.

Once in class, Ohno said, "Be your own ashes," and he sat and observed his students for two hours, perfectly still.

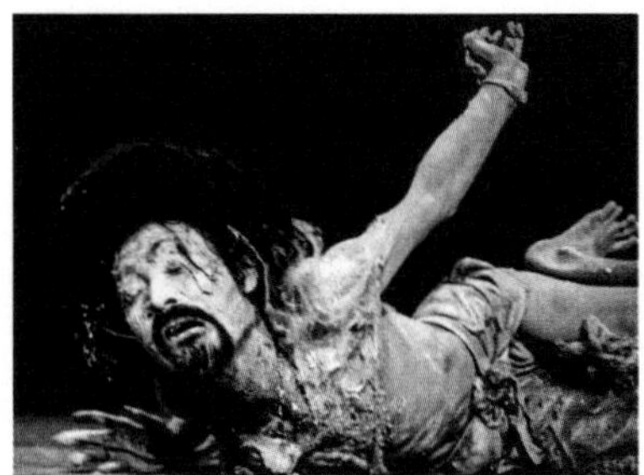

This is the self destroyed: Tatsumi Hijikata.

The End of Pretend

Meanwhile, in downtown New York, where the war was not a visceral, embodied experience, some choreographers moved away from articulated meaning toward form, inviting content to emerge through the forms themselves.

Merce Cunningham radically moved the gaze to the horizon line. This decision in his choreography cannot be overemphasized. By centering the lifted chest and eyes, which were once fixed on the heavens or deep inside, he crashed through psychology and obliterated romanticism in dance. Although he held onto the body's ballet line, he rejected many things about modern dance and ballet; he dismissed centralized space, hierarchical phrasing, the placement of the torso, implicit morality, and any distinct connection to music. For Cunningham, movement itself was the subject matter, not the afterlife, suffering, or any moral question. The self is no self. But the work is not selfless; the actions of the body, the body as self, became the subject matter. As early as the late 1940s, Cunningham handed decision-making to the universe by implementing chance techniques, and in this act, he paradoxically embraced a new form of choreographic decision-making. Chance operations—a nonauthorial, algorithmic pose of objectivity—define the work. His elegant, intellectual, ongoing experiment collaborated with the gods of chance.

He said, "We give ourselves away at every moment; we do not, therefore, have to try to do it."

Simultaneously, George Balanchine

On the giant stage of the New York City Ballet, the great Russian choreographer George Balanchine revolutionized ballet with pure, clean abstraction. Uptown, Balanchine was considering some of the same compositional and nontheatrical ideas that Cunningham was considering downtown: the deconstruction and poetics of action itself. In his neoclassical ballets, dancers look straight ahead, perform non-narrative movement, and exit and enter the stage by simply walking. Although temperamentally cool, in Balanchine's hands, these pedestrian motifs hold an ardent artistry that registered as pure passion, creating an artistic rather than personal heat. Like Cunningham, through his full embrace of what *is*, via the rigor of presence itself, Balanchine trafficked in "the mysteries" of dance that live entirely outside narrative analysis.

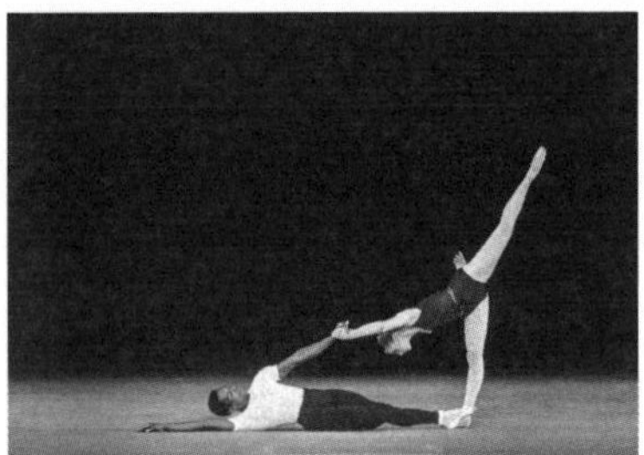

Balanchine's *Agon* (1957)

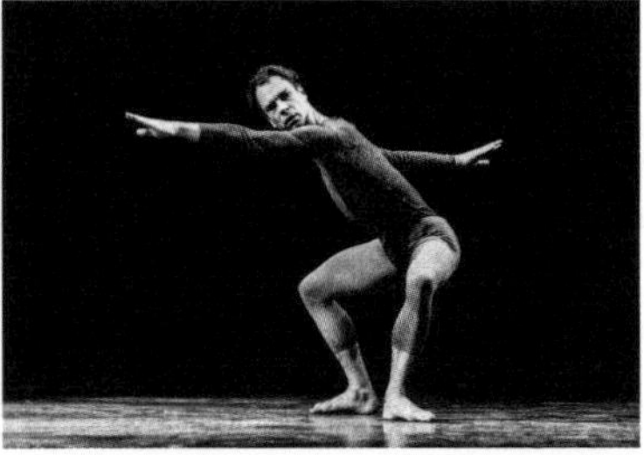

Cunningham's *Changeling* (1957)

Generations in dance
are short when the
world is exploding

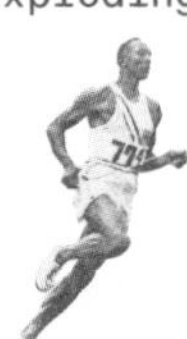

Dailiness: The Dancer Is People

Only a few years later, in the early 1960s, the Judson Church movement emerged from the shadow of another war, Vietnam. There was a chill in the air, a distrust of the notion that angst and suffering are noble, as well as a distrust of pure form. The choreographers of the Judson Church pivoted to embrace the pedestrian and the quotidian. Suspicious of virtuosity and its hierarchy, they created a new virtuosity out of the everyday. Simple daily tasks were put onstage, and these non-theatrical choices became the new theatrical. Though fiercely individualistic, these choreographers collectively translated the ordinary into the sublime. Expressing Vietnam-era disillusionment and directly rejecting the very notion of authority, their movement vocabulary and phrasing became nonhierarchical. Walking across the room had more currency than a triple pirouette. Costumes became street clothes, sets became the room, and dancers became people.

Satisfyin' Lover (1967) is a postmodern dance by Steve Paxton.

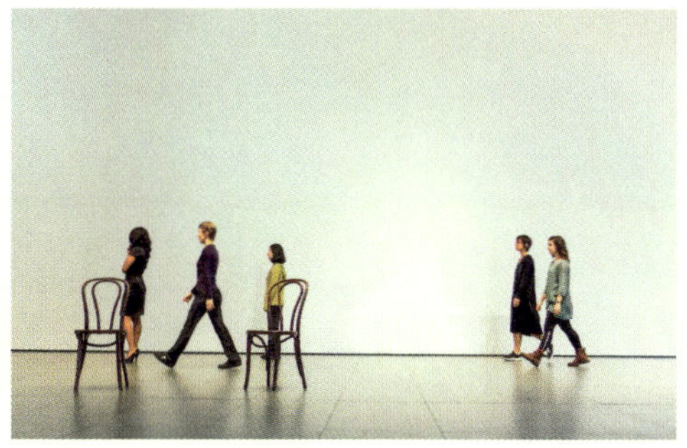

This dance is about the day.

The dance writer Jill Johnston rejected the subjectivity of Cunningham's algorithmic objectivity in favor of the chaos and sweat of living underground as the "second sex." Brilliantly conflating her roles as journalist and performer, Johnston unapologetically and without polish argued, ranted, and preened; her tonality crashed into male power structures. She was unabashedly and intentionally out of control on both the stage and the page, and she performed her role(s) with vital intellectual rigor. Johnston's "self" wasn't an algorithm or an ordered version of randomness; it was the complex, imperfect disarray of life.

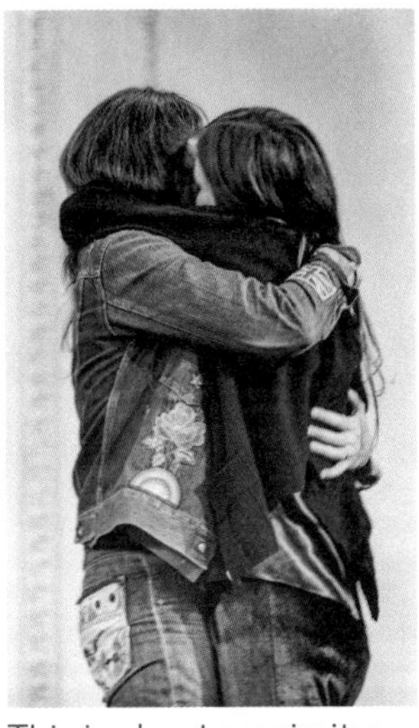

This is about proximity: female bodies in space.

*Authorial pause
of space and time.
I sit down in a
downtown dance
theater in NYC
in 1980.

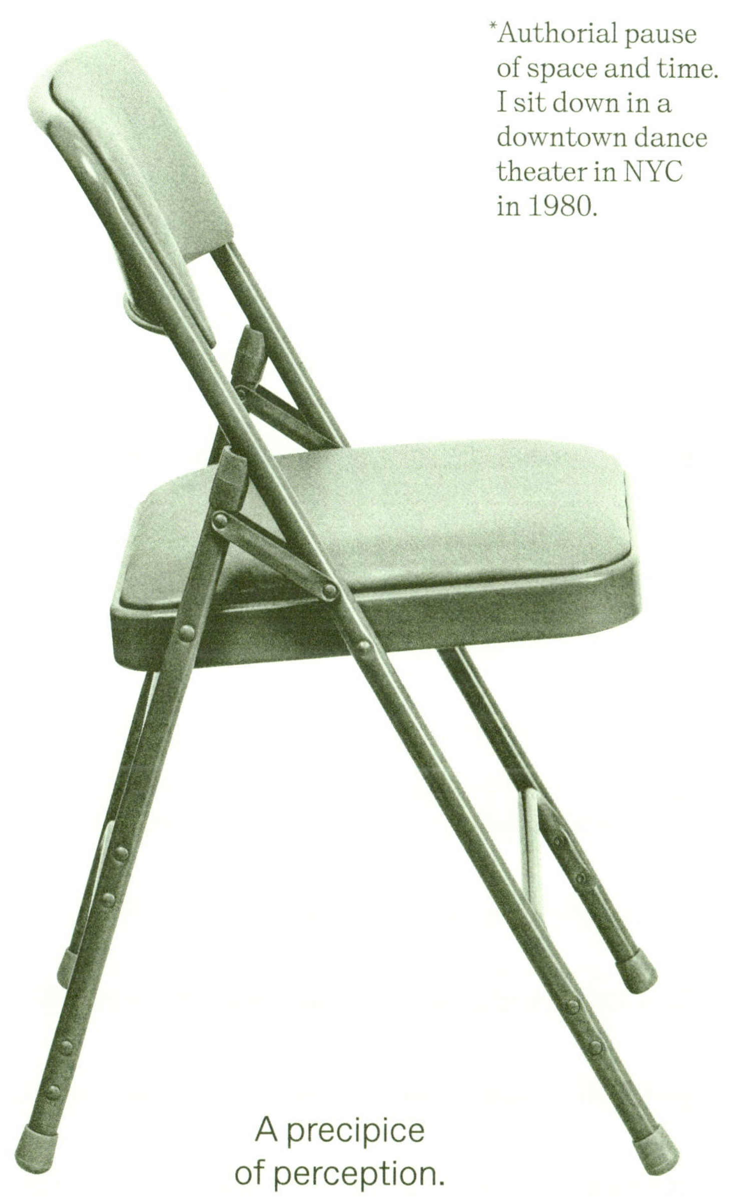

A precipice
of perception.

Reagan in the Drinking Water

In the 1980s, Reaganism offered (some) Americans a new form of delusion, a free pass to live large and buy extravagantly. But there was little to have or to get in New York City's downtown dance world. Emerging NYC choreographers of this period had grown up when the art marketplace saw dance as unnecessary and society viewed dance as suspect. Artistically, we (when I say "we" or "us" here, I am talking about a *very* loose group of choreographers working downtown in experimental dance in NYC in the 1980s) were focused on a dance world outside of that marketplace, a space devoted to experimentation. I didn't know anyone who toured or had a "career." Our horizon line was largely Dance Theater Workshop, Danspace Project, the Kitchen, and Performance Space 122. Class was cheap, rent was cheap, and studios were cheap. We went to a daily ballet class; many of us studied with Zvi Gothiener, who taught ballet in hiking boots. Zvi centered the gaze and neutralized the spine's relationship to the pelvis, changing the tone and muscularity of ballet without altering the vocabulary or the sequencing. We took class six days a week; although ballet didn't overtly influence our work, it was our secret training, sewn into our choreography. The discipline of ballet informed the rigor of our investigations. In every piece we made and watched, the bar was set high for nothing less than a formal dismantling of everything. Our sole criterion was gigantic: we were looking for—demanding—some slight shift in the form of dance itself.

Though we had elected to work and live under the radar, downtown dance had its own hierarchies of power and authority. Like our immediate forbearers, the Judson Church choreographers, we rejected structures of authority in our dances. But the Judson Church choreographers operated as a collective and used an empty gym for a stage, while we were all competing for gigs and inadequate commissions in the downtown theaters. In effect, we were tacitly accepting the power structures of our small world—naively supporting them by infusing them with the power of our artistry, which the gatekeepers needed to do their business. This was a problematic relationship with the culture we were critiquing. It was a market of supply and demand, and that equation was always against us: there was too much supply and very little demand. How often have I sat in the audience of Performance Space 122 or the Kitchen and mused on the fact that we dance artists both supplied the goods and, as audience members, consumed those goods? On the one hand, we were subordinate to the theater gatekeepers, allowing them to cheaply appropriate our labor and ideas for their own gain and prestige; on the other, we had actively chosen a life outside of the mainstream dance world, a life without a ladder to climb to stability, so as to practice unbounded experimentation. We perceived ourselves as free, but we were not.

New York City, 1984: What I Saw

The first piece I saw by the Wooster Group was *LSD (...Just the High Points...)*, directed by Elizabeth LeCompte in 1984, and watching it put me in an art stupor. I went back to see it countless times to try to make sense of what I was seeing, but no matter how earnestly I worked to detach myself as I studied *LSD*, I remained in a blissful state of confusion. In retrospect, my disorientation was warranted. LeCompte was deeply committed to ripping up all the contracts directors have ever (implicitly) signed with their audiences.

This dizzying masterpiece simultaneously changed so many formal art games for me. Like the many subsequent Wooster Group pieces I later witnessed, *LSD* operated more as visual art in that the surface of the work (set and sound design, staging, objects, and costumes) had more meaning than story or psychology. From a storytelling perspective, there was and was not a narrative; I experienced narrative as buried under living itself. Played out in real time through an aesthetic of the quotidian, there was a sense that the performers were living on stage, and any narrative was less important than this living. And here, for the first time, I saw multiple televisions for purposes of abstraction, a directorial choice that made undeniable the ubiquity of this glowing object in the rooms of our lives. The monitors functioned to layer reality, not to clarify it. And the piece introduced live feed to theater. With live feed, LeCompte both decentralized the space and activated the offstage. I could see the performers being taped live in the offstage/upstage-right position, but in a nod to the contemporary exponential self, I also saw them on the video monitors, which were rolled on tracks up and down the raked stage accompanied by loud and dissociative machinery sounds. The radically kinetic staging was like that of a panel discussion, but it was also Kabuki-like in its particular respect for form. The shape and positioning of the body itself were mined as a compositional element. And for the first time, I saw microphones on stage; LeCompte exploited them for their extreme tones, affects, and volumes. She embroidered the amplified text into an aural landscape of music and literal sound effects, often wittily reassigning sounds to unrelated actions. Eschewing long-established ideas about motivation in acting, the Wooster Group actors didn't perform traditional dramatic "beats" but instead seemed to find zones of emotion, which, like weather, existed for periods of time; here, the language felt as if it were undressed. Even the frame of her works, their first and last moments, were reimagined. In rejecting the "curtain up, curtain down" tradition, LeCompte's pieces seemed to illegibly trail on and off, leaving me beautifully unmoored on both ends.

And the dances...The dances would erupt perfectly and unexpectedly out of moments in the complex aural scores. I always thought that the same dances were performed from piece to piece, as if the company had a folk-dance tradition all its own that I could watch forever, binding me to them through their dances.

All this sounds very formal, but the effect was the opposite. When the performance illegibly dissipated, I always found myself bathed in emotion, and this sentiment was coming from my art heart in response to the brilliance of the artistry. I experienced the work as life-affirming, as visceral evidence that in the hands of a few and in ways that are radical and uncanny, form itself can shift to express who we are, and we, in turn, can be altered in its midst. This refraction-and-loop structure was the subject matter for me; it was, in effect, my church.

In those days, I didn't see choreographers in the audience at the Wooster Group; it seemed to me that the downtown dance and theater worlds were inexplicably separated. Only much later, when their televisions, microphones, and sound cues began to seep into the dance world, did I see the Wooster Group's heavy influence on form and surface spread through downtown dance.

And concurrently, in 1984, I saw Pina Bausch's large-scale theatrical choreography as it traveled from Germany to New York for the first time. Contrary to what was going on in dance in the United States, Bausch created a world rather than revealed our world. Bausch rejected the minimalism, the formalism, and the mundane that so fascinated American choreographers in favor of the highly theatrical. In her work, there were no pedestrian bodies in sweatpants and T-shirts performing tasks on stage. Her dancers wore slips, evening gowns, high heels, and suits, and the work had an aroma of the post–World War II era rather than of post-Vietnam. The tone was sardonic and urbane as she theatricalized societal customs and behaviors. In Bausch's wry, cosmopolitan worlds, men and women fought and cried in repetitive loops and often talked with the audience. What interested me was that Bausch engaged with the pleasures of theater—but without the narrative. Her concerns included relationships, character, circumstance, costume, dialogue, and social dance, and these elements were manipulated using choreographic tools. The work was durational, lasting late into the evening, a trippy and elegant party with complicated, intelligent guests—a party to remember your entire life.

The 1980s: Six New York City Dance Makers Who Shifted the Form Forward in My Beginner's Mind

Bill T. Jones and Arnie Zane dance *Blauvelt Mountain.* Deceptively simple, tonally calm, and coolly personal, *Blauvelt Mountain* addresses their hallowed relationality through compositional elements. Crafting motion, time, and shape, they express their duality. *Blauvelt Mountain* holds an art-making elegance that speaks to social justice, love, and the power of two bodies in space.

Bebe Miller, light and disciplined, invents in real time an original vocabulary with abstraction set against real life. Her phrases are discursive movement sentences that never end up where we think they are going. And Miller's performance possesses a charm you can't learn but must be born with—a dance charm. Both intimate and distant, her work is deeply tied to New York City, her city, telling us through this cosmopolitan complexity where she comes from and is going at once.

Tere O'Connor introduces a new virtuosity of brazenly arcane technique to the stage. In a firm rejection of articulated meaning, he dazzles with long phrases and new ideas of dissonance as harmony. While I watch his work, which to me is one long piece, I think about friendship as a kind of love that takes the form of artistry.

In his landmark dance *THEM,* Ishmael Houston-Jones melds disenfranchisement and community with a ritual slaughter. The first time I see it, I am too stunned to know what has happened to me. Though I am terrified, I return for a second time to study and digest his voice, a new intersection of physical abstraction and politics.

With a virtuosity and emotional intelligence for choreographic formality, Blondell Cummings vaults considerations like gesture and repetition into issues of Black female portraiture. She bravely brings character to an atmosphere of pure abstraction and detachment; her subject is family, the world she came from, so rarely seen on these stages. The materiality of her work is the domestic—a paper bag, a frying pan. Using simple physical actions, she employs the vocabulary of task-based work to reveal the interiority of characters on stages heretofore devoted to pure form. Her choreography ranges from the large-scale and cinematic to the quotidian in an instant. Cummings's choreography: inspiration, aspiration, respiration.

RoseAnne Spradlin snatches the female gaze with both hands and throws it back at you, daring you to grapple with it. Her ugly is gorgeous; her dances have at once gravity and gravitas. In a female argument with Cunningham's lines and algorithms, Spradlin's shapes are bulbous, bumpy, dripping, and oozing. Spradlin both destroys and galvanizes by embracing the totality of the female body in ways seen before only by such artists as Lucien Freud and Louise Bourgeois. Her choreographic gaze shocks me into remembering who I am, who I came from, and who I can be.

When the news cycle accelerates, so do dance forms

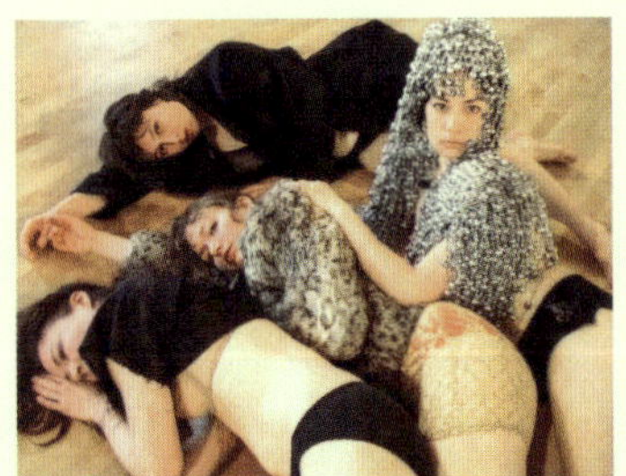

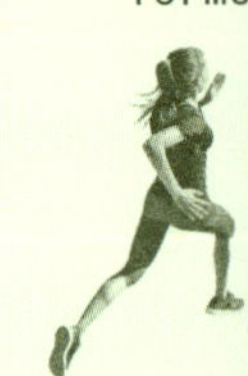

Reagan's America Doesn't End in 1988

With so much going wrong in the twentieth century, dance bridges into the twenty-first with a searing distrust of authority and form. Immediately after Donald Trump's election in 2016, who dances and who is danced for are urgent subject matter. In a powerful response to the horror of electing someone so openly racist and sexist, New York's downtown dance world responds by finally shining a light onto underrepresented voices and bodies of color onstage. Dance artists are making dances about the profound dimensional implications of this belated invitation. These dances appear at once communal and very private. Framed by shock, they are immediate call-and-responses to and with the world. Dance matters again. Even in the smallest of theaters, the import is giant.

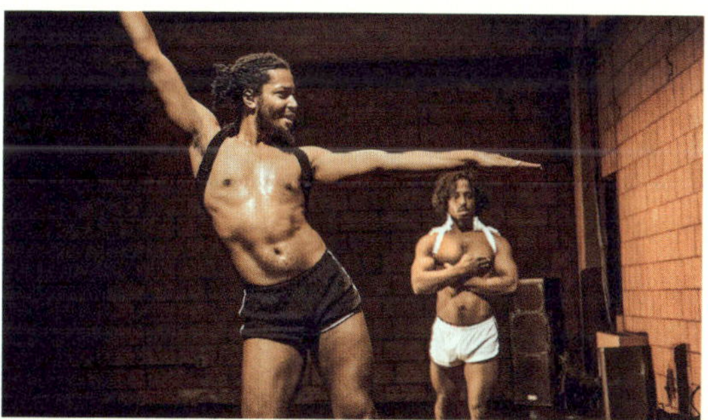

This is Mankini's body in space.

The Body in Virtual Space: COVID-19 Dances, 2020

Issues of the pedestrian body in public space are parsed and governed for the first time. Social choreographies are now a matter of life and death. Choreographic elements are in the news: proximity, time, space, duets, and group gatherings. The simplest physical actions are in focus: how close we stand is scrutinized, how to greet someone is reimagined, how to pass someone on the street, how to take a walk—all these actions are dynamic. We can no longer hand things to one another, shake, hug, converse, or gather. The movement of all our bodies must follow and invent new choreographic directives.

Our very breath, our saliva, our sweat is suddenly meaningful. The power of the body is suddenly very present.

Presence itself is in question.

This is a choreographic structure in North Brunswick, New Jersey, on a Thursday in March 2020 based on verticality, proximity, and stillness.

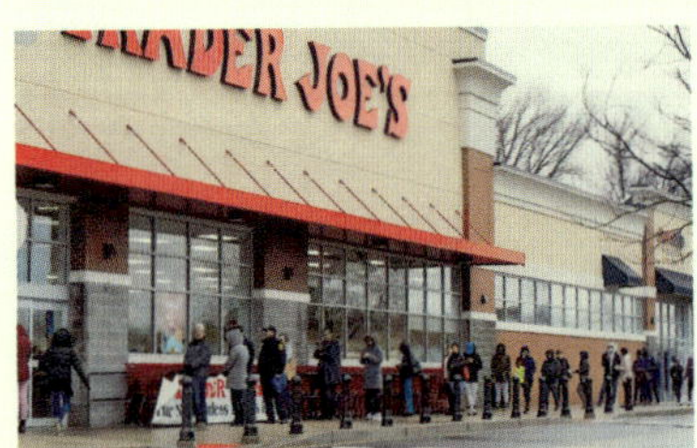

This line is a choreography of six-foot separation.

The Poetics of Zoom

In March 2020, days after the COVID-19 lockdown, theaters and studios are shuttered. By necessity, the virtual performance space emerges as the dominant place to see dance. These quick inventions speak to the essential, primal need to dance. The visceral and the virtual conflate.

If we felt ourselves moving closer to an online life before COVID, now dancers fully move their stage to the computer screen. The embodied form is disembodied as an image of the body situated firmly in virtual space.

Stuck at home with the choreographic directive to "shelter in place," dance makers look for cheap and accessible stages.

The online platform Zoom becomes a quick solution to the dancer's inability to get sweaty in a studio with other dancers. The structure of Zoom, with its neat, symmetrical staging and physical directives, invites choreographers to explore its algorithms. It's so choreographic, really: a geometric, poetic form with implicit limitations. Even the choreographic decision of duration is part of its poetics; Zoom turns off abruptly after forty minutes—if you didn't buy the prime membership.

House lights: GO.

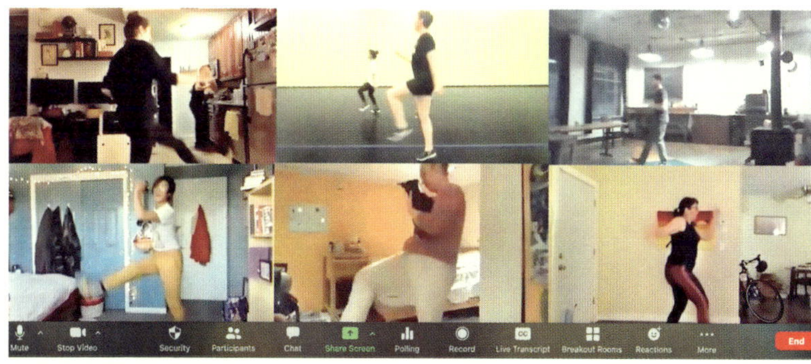

These are disembodied bodies on Zoom.

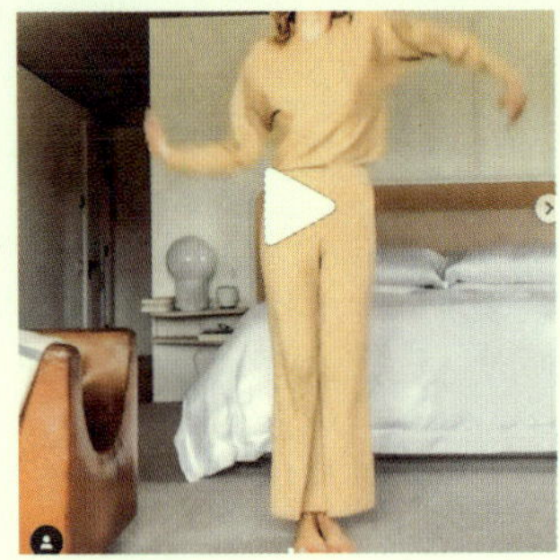

This is a domestic folk-dance form: TikTok.

Since dance is an especially organic and mutable form, I think about how it was impacted over the long-term by this virus. While we were inside and essentially in solos and duets with intense physical restrictions, our dances became small domestic kinesphere compositions, more intimate, rough, and shorter in duration.

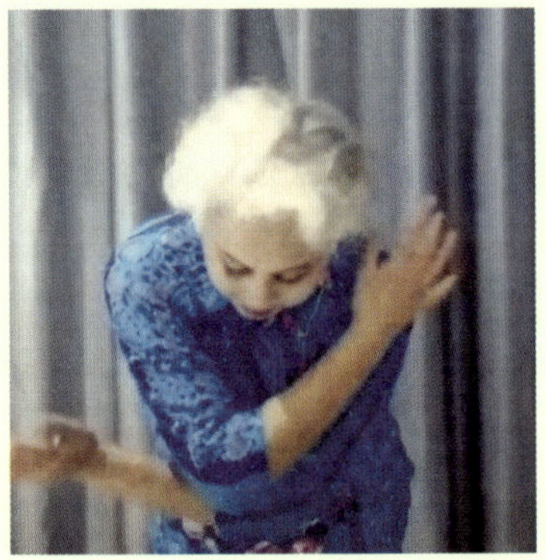

This is a dance from home.

Consider someone who aesthetically organizes their body's actions into a dance and then performs and posts it on social media as part of the evolution of the form.

During COVID, the nurses in the ER break out in dance.

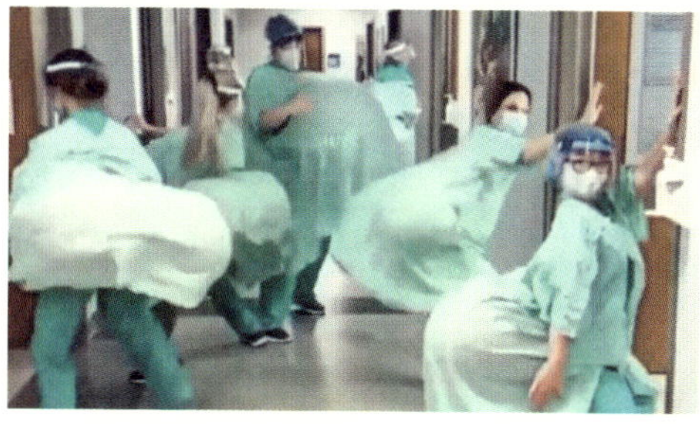

Ecstatic dancing goes back to the beginnings of why we danced.

~~The End.~~

I was about to write "The End,"
but dance is too live, too fundamental,
too dynamic to write those words.

Because as you read this,
someone is making a dance right now,
someone is teaching someone a dance right now.

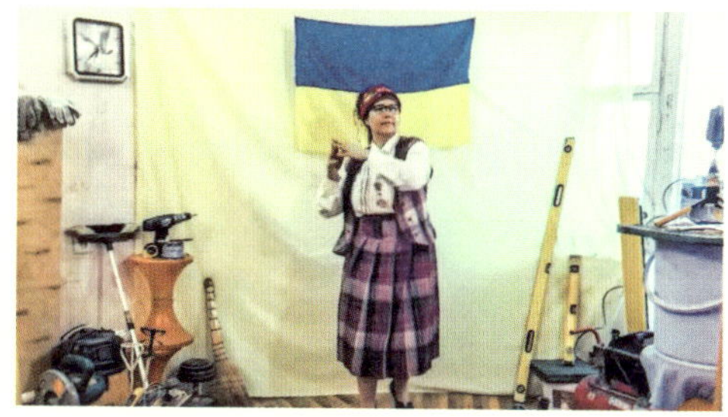

Someone is just dancing somewhere right now.

Dancing is living.

Page 2 (top): Japanese cranes' courtship duet. Image: iStock/plusphoto
Page 2 (bottom): The Gela Painter, attributed, detail of Panathenaic prize amphora, Benghazi, Libya, 333–332 BCE. British Museum, London
Page 3 (top): Hellenistic statuette, 3rd century BCE. Metropolitan Museum of Art, New York
Page 3 (bottom): Bas-relief of Corybants' war dance (Neo-Attic after Athenian relief from the fourth century BCE), first century. Vatican Museum
Page 4 (center): Acheloös Painter, attributed, amphora (Greek), c. 520 BCE. Metropolitan Museum of Art, New York
Page 6 (top): Ambrogio Lorenzetti, detail of the Allegory of Good and Bad Government, 1338–39. Palazzo Pubblico, Siena
Page 6 (bottom): image: Folk Arts Center of New England
Page 7 (top): Morris Dancers in the Westminster Day of Dance 2009, Trafalgar Square, May 9, 2009. Photo © urban75
Page 7 (bottom): Sandro Botticelli, detail of *Annunciation*, c. 1490. Glasgow Museums Collection, Glasgow, Scotland
Page 8 (top): Giovanni di Paolo, *Five Angels Dancing*, c. 1430. Musée Condé, Chantilly, Oise, France
Page 8 (bottom): WCCC runners, 1912. Library of Congress, Washington, DC
Page 9 (top): Ellen Price as La Sylphide, 1903. Photo by Peter Elfelt
Page 10: Dancers in Oskar Schlemmer's *Triadic Ballet* (1912) at the Metropol, Berlin, 1926. Photo by Ernst Schneider
Page 11: Martha Graham in *Lamentation* (1930). Photo by Herta Moselsio, c. 1939
Page 12 (top): Drawing by Annie-B Parson on photocopy
Page 12 (bottom): Sophie Taeuber-Arp and her sister, Erika Schlegel, in Hopi Native American–themed costumes designed by the artist, 1922. Photographer unknown
Page 13 (top): Illustration from Henry Gray's *Gray's Anatomy*, illustrated by Henry Vandyke Carter, 1858
Page 13 (bottom): Louis Zamperini, who represented the United States in the 1936 Olympics, Berlin
Page 14: Butoh dancer and choreographer Hijikata Tatsumi, 1972. Photo by Onozuka Makoto Hijikata
Page 16 (left): New York City Ballet dancers Arthur Mitchell and Suzanne Farrell in George Balanchine's *Agon* (1957), 1963. Photo by Jack Mitchell
Page 16 (right): Merce Cunningham in *Changeling*, 1957. Photo by Richard Rutledge
Page 16 (bottom): Jesse Owens at the 1936 Olympics, Berlin
Page 17: Steve Paxton's *Satisfying Lover* (1967), performed at the Museum of Modern Art, New York, 2012. Photo by Julieta Cervantes
Page 18: Jill Johnston and an unidentified woman embracing onstage during "A Dialogue on Women's Liberation," Town Hall, New York, April 30, 1971. Photo by Fred W. McDarrah, © Fred W. McDarrah/MUUS Collection
Page 26 (left): Rebecca Serrell Cyr, Natalie Green, Rebecca Wender, and Molly Poerstel in RoseAnne Spradlin's *beginning of something*, 2011. Photo by RoseAnne Spradlin
Page 27 (top): Makini (jumatatu m. poe) and Jermone Donte Beacham, *Let 'im Move You: A Study* (2013/2016) and *Let 'im Move You: This Is a Success*, 2016. Photo by Ian Douglas
Page 28: Image Patti Sapone/NJ Advance Media
Page 29 (bottom): Restaging for the small screen(s) by Elizabeth DeMent of Annie-B Parson's *The Snow Falls in the Winter*, Sarah Lawrence Dance Program Performance Project, Zoom performance, spring 2020
Page 31 (top): adrienneporter0 on TikTok

Every effort has been made to trace copyright holders for the use of copyrighted material. The publisher apologizes for any errors or omissions and would be grateful if notified of corrections that should be incorporated in future editions of this book.

It's about pretending, really. Or becoming, changing, in order to invite the rains, conquer the enemy, call the sun, attract the mate, fly. First is the urge, the need, to gather strength, to charge the situation, love, stride toward, leave behind whatever hasn't been enough just now or just before. To take on the rains is to humble yourself before a greater power.

Then, Form. It blooms, the slightest shift between what you are and what is needed to invite the enemy, conquer the rains, slide toward the mate, be the sun, soar above all. Soar. And then again, tomorrow, next season, bloom again, take shape, take time, take form, become force, become necessary. Become light, the energy, the sun, the partner, the kinfolk. Become again. The first time is an accident; only the first time is free. Recall, reuse, reinvent, remember. Much later, Form becomes the rite, becomes the dance, becomes the next best, the best approximate, the pretending sun. Never the Sun.

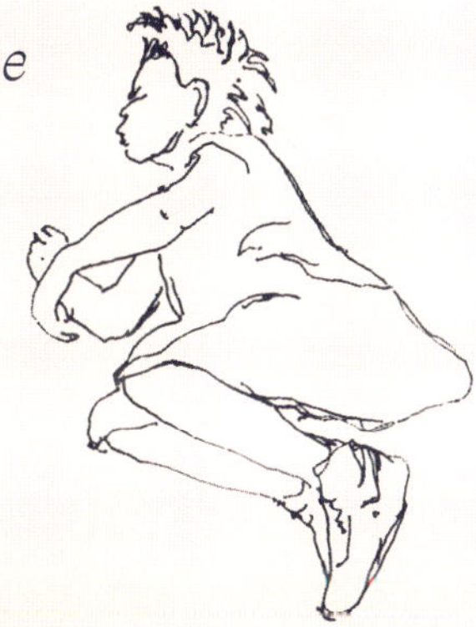

+++

Dancing is personal. It's inside of you. How else to talk about it? We all have it, this forming of the world, noting how the world moves and takes its time. We imitate the action that catches our eye; we try on the walk, the stride. We want to be able to call the sun, so we watch to see how it's done. Every material carries its own angle of repose, sorted by granular specifics: the way we rest our heads and hips, curve our spines, waiting for the *dream move* to strike. The information inside seeps outward to guide how we place our body and self in relation to… everything. Every dance carries its own angle of projection, aimed toward connection and deliverance, in answer to what seems necessary; in gratitude for what has come to pass; and, of course, because it is so outrageously fun to do. Yes! At some point, some folk lose faith in their ability to conjure and are left to demonstrate their magic rather than inhabit it or ask the conjurer/dance maker to work their voodoo instead. It's a soulful practice, a mindfulness that begins before we have the words to describe it. Our feet press the ground, moving us forward one step at a time. We note the weight of the spirits we carry on our backs, whether they've decided to lift us or forgive us. Our arms reach. Our hips tilt and wreck, generating a certainty that rises into our throats and into our eyes. We command, we are commanded, we contain multitudes, we twist and shout.

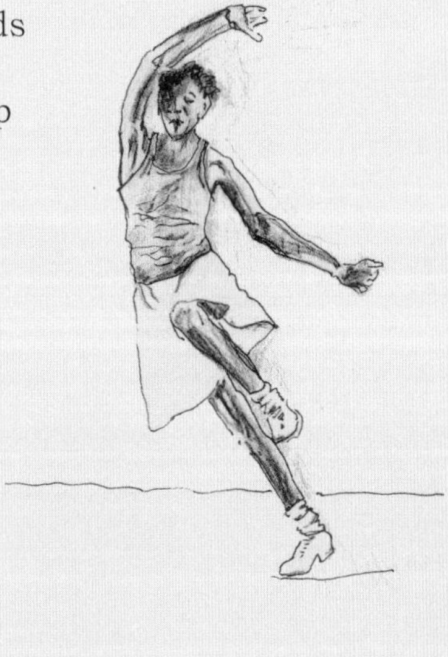

+++

There's a practice here. Our teachers position us to receive the information, and we all wait to see if we've been heard. The first teacher shapes the ground in ways that are magical. She teaches you how to whittle the space surrounding you so that you can glide through a texture no one else can see. My first teacher also taught me how to whittle a stick and the name of the tree it came from, but that's another story. Another teacher asks you to become an empty chocolate box (for real! He did!), and you do. And once you've become that empty box or that flight of clouds or that warrior, you carry enough of a trace to reenter that space, to become that beat, to become whatever wasn't there before.

A short while ago, I watched a group of young women on a stage form a circle, backs facing outward, arms interlaced. Their heads dipped down, looking inward while sensing the whole of them breathing. They were about to begin an excerpt from Martha Graham's *Steps in the Street*, from the larger work *Chronicle*, more than eighty years after it was first performed. They had learned this work, coached by teachers and elders, the same way many of us have learned how to enter form. Attuned to the *becoming*. Taking on a previous era's necessity, making it their own. Graham's work was choreographed in the 1930s as a response to the rise of Fascism in Europe, and these women I watched found their own extremely current way to transform the somatic into the political.

They did just fine. I believed in their dancing;
I believed them.

For centuries (eons?), we've spiraled through styles of moving, returning to and then retooling our bodies, taking on the task of speaking the old dances, the new fun, crafting the technical skill and whizbang, shaping force and emotion into what we need to know about how we need to live. We are guided by the particulars we choose as focal points. We follow the truth of our moment in time. I say this to tell you where I'm coming from, which is necessary to tell you how dancing happens. How it happened for me is just one trace among many, of course, but it's the one I know well enough to make me pause and check: How does that work? How does it move, really?

I'm a New Yorker, raised in the Red Hook Houses, Brooklyn. I've lived in New York for much of my life, and for most of it, I've danced in some form or another. I've been a pedestrian, a schoolgirl, a reader, an audience member, a friend of friends who dance and make dances, a Black woman, a neighbor, a sister. Because of the gravitational pull of so many kinds of people moving together all at once, we know how New York entices dancers and makers to enter its orbit. The rub between the forms we practice generates our cultural fascia, our internal maps of enthrallment.

As a teen, then a twenty-, thirty-, forty-something in the city, I grew into my own habit of the choreographic, the syntactical, the rhythmical. My own manner of noting action and context stems from the pace of growing up native, being *from* a neighborhood as opposed to living in one. One's culture is a strategy, a system of appetite and appropriation. The assortment of stuff to navigate is bewildering until the ground tilts to guide you, and gravity arranges the flotsam in time with what you can perceive.

When I was growing up and navigating the city, the subway was the ground level—mappable. When my mother wanted her children to *know things*, she would find free concerts and ice-skating rinks and libraries and know which train to take and where to stand when the doors opened. She would do what was necessary to find the singular experiences that set the tone of the questions we would later ask.

When my mother wanted to give her children the leg up she saw other people give theirs, she found Henry Street Settlement, an institution on the Lower East Side established in the late nineteenth century to provide social services, the arts, and opportunities for immigrant families. Her children had classes in art and music and, at the Henry Street Playhouse, dance classes taught by members of Alwin Nikolais's Playhouse Dance Company. (Years later, Murray Louis, my teacher at Henry Street and a modern-dance icon, sits with me in a hotel lobby in Los Angeles; both of our companies are there on tour. He tells me to remember to be gracious with our curtain calls. I listen to Murray; he's speaking to me as, if not quite an equal, then an elder. I listen, somewhere between grown-self-in-charge and child-self-entranced. It doesn't occur to me that this is as special a moment for him as for me.)

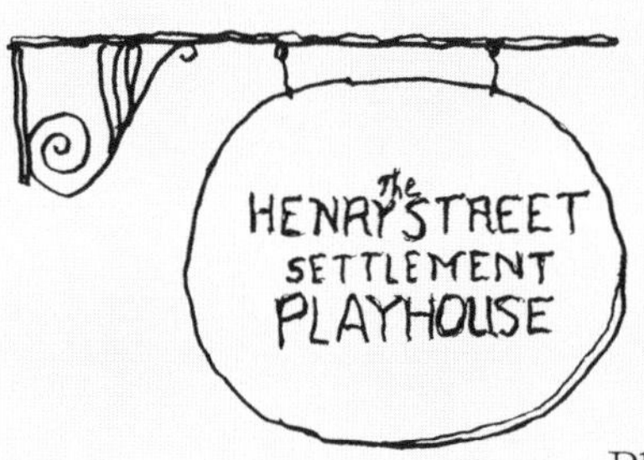

The journey to Henry Street, from our own Smith-Ninth Street subway station to the East Broadway stop on the Lower East Side, involved emerging upward into a landscape that blossomed out of dark tunnels into unfamiliar arrangements of people and place. We'd arrive without crossing the land, without seeing the East River change according to the weather. We never felt Chinatown vibrating a block behind us as we walked through the Jewish Orthodox neighborhood.

Traveling from northwest Brooklyn with its waterfront and narrow single-family houses along the edge of the docks, we knew the shift of activity and populace that marked our arrival: the Hasidim and Latin folk shopping together at the Essex Street Market (sawdust-covered floor, my mother buying chicken carcasses and spices cheaper than at our A&P); my discovery of Bleecker Street cafés; the boom boxes next to the continual basketball game at the West Fourth Street station; the thrill of available cash in the crowds at Thirty-Fourth Street and Macy's/Gimbels/Franklin Simon (a great store, sold wonderful shoes); the expanded air around Rockefeller Center, Seventh Avenue, Carnegie Hall, Town Hall.

Pablo Casals at Town Hall, alone onstage with his cello: we watch him from the highest balcony, then head home by subway, so late at night, my brother and sister and me falling asleep, my mother keeping watch.

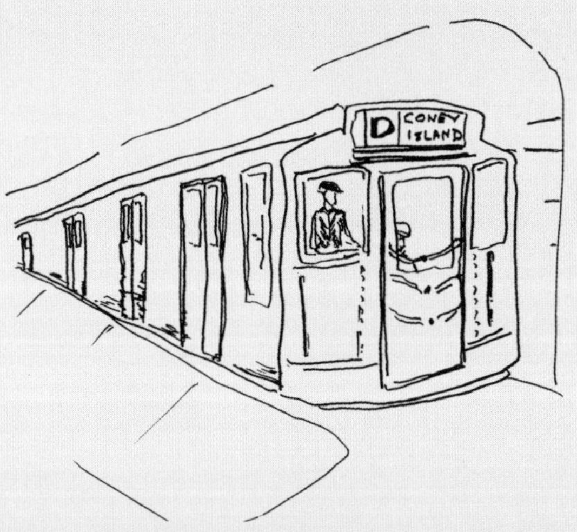

The days contain trips to the Donnell Library branch, the Museum of Modern Art (never called MoMA), the re-Blackening past Fifty-Ninth Street into Harlem and beyond. The Twister floor plan of racial, musical, economic, and inspirational diversity that shapes the city seemed sharper then, but that's what memory does.

1. *Stand to wait for the D train at Smith-Ninth Street station on Saturday mornings (third car from the front, second set of doors, ready to exit through the doors opposite at the East Broadway stop).*

2. *Always walk the shortest possible distance anywhere you need to go.*

3. *Do not stroll, do not wander; go directly to your destination, except on trips to Schirmer's on Forty-Ninth Street for piano sheet music; in that particular case, take all the time you need.*

4. *Avoid the Bronx. Avoid the Gowanus projects. Avoid the Fort Hamilton Parkway subway stop in Brooklyn—full of ghosts.*

5. *Note how Black folk in Harlem differ from Black folk in Brooklyn, much less Queens; no need to discuss.*

6. *Note the days when New York City is yours to define, which are most days.*

If we're lucky and the timing is right, at some point we loosen our grip on the singularity of our own experience as emblematic of the world and embrace the range of what is possible. When we choose dance, the world first contracts and then expands. The pulse entices us: the simplicity of right step to left, the countershift through the body, the swing of the jump rope *just so*, skipping the beat, cooling the body style, feet close to the ground, then airborne. Or we're enticed by an unfamiliar timing that frames an ordinary shift of weight, so much so that a gesture seems to include all our collected memories, embodied and lodged, with no words to explain the situation.

+++

THINGS THAT HAPPEN WHEN THE TIMING IS RIGHT

Bebe Miller

What follows is a timetable of sorts—incomplete, of course, as it's mostly mine and I'm still here. But it's a chance to place certain markers in relationship to one another. Hindsight is helpful, though imperfect. Much of what I recall has a flattened perspective that's not at all photographic; I remember remembering. Over time, events thicken and refer more deeply to their original context, more than I was first able to perceive. This seems reason enough; I wait for what I remember to show up.

Imagine this: a swarm of ways of moving in the city that feed the choices one makes to dance in the city. These tight whirls of *place*—the stoop, the downtown loft, the uptown theater, the street—attract their audience, the other practitioners of the form.

My level of skill as a young double Dutch rope jumper (intermediate—could hold my own) gave me a certain set of chops that circuitously linked me to Balkan folk dancing and West African dance a decade later (intermediate—could hold my own). Ten years after that, the accumulated references of coolness, dynamic analysis on the fly (what is that *thing* they're doing, and why does it move that way?), the various cultural/political signifiers that spoke at different volumes and with distinct intentions—all of these have taken on the form of the Very Large Array of Influence.[1] I receive this information chronologically; while it is determined by when I show up and at which stoop, loft, theater, or street, it may best be imagined as an experiential progression through small revelations, nudging me toward my own self, the one who dances.

The phenomenon of contemporary dance in New York City, its currency in downtown and uptown scenes, is a training ground for twenty-somethings on the lookout for ways to

1 The Very Large Array Radio Telescope is a big set of dish antennae precisely aimed toward the cosmos from Socorro, New Mexico. The VLA of Influence is less specific.

belong. There are distinctions to be made over which concerts or classes you gravitate to; where you show up is witnessed and subtle adjustments in relevance are chalked up. We dance.

1960. What feels like happenstance to a child often transpires from clear choices made by a mother with a plan. A group of family photos feature my siblings and me in assorted costumes for various children's dances at Henry Street Playhouse. We were bags of gold from the above-the-clouds section of "Jack and the Beanstalk," three fat birds who eat Hansel and Gretel's trail of breadcrumbs, and the strings of the lyre Orpheus plays to charm Hades and rescue Eurydice. Participating in these events was a given at Henry Street, part of growing up in the city. Where you were taken as a kid was where things happened before you grew into making choices on your own.

Raymond Johnson was Orpheus. He was three years older (a lifetime!), old enough to have chosen, as a tall, medium-brown Black gay teenager in the 1950s, to explore the abstract kinetics of Nikolais's *tensile involvement* of space, time, and motion. And then later, as a dancer with both the Nikolais Dance Theatre and Murray Louis Dance Company, Raymond signaled there might be a possible life in dancing. For several years, we were at the same summer camp. I remember him working on a solo involving a rocking chair that pitched forward into an upturned garbage-can lid, noisy and abrupt. It was a choice that I couldn't envision myself making. It was a choice outside the realm of what I could *feel*. It was a kind of dancing with no reference to steps or phrasing, to any of my teachers. I didn't have the tools to recognize what he was doing or to conceive of how his outsider art was beginning to take shape. "A dancer who was both sensuous and impish," according to his 1987 obituary.[2] He died at forty from "complications" (AIDS, perhaps), having disbanded his own company seven years prior.

2 "Raymond Johnson, 40; Dancer-Choreographer," *New York Times*, March 28, 1987.

Raymond was privy to a way of living inside of art making that was unavailable to me. So much depends on the kindness of teachers and parents, let alone strangers, to suggest a way to work against apparent limitations. Or better, a way to work while keeping the assumed restrictions in your periphery: keep an eye out but go on and play. And then, how best to wander: Away from what's assumed? Toward a retelling of what's been there all along?

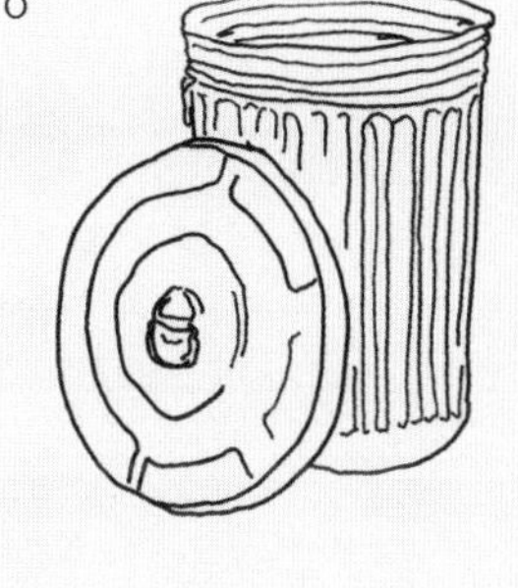

It's helpful to realize that parts of us travel under our skin, arrive by happenstance, take their time to manifest, collide, and then show up.

1966. It's my junior year in high school. My friend Marcus and I dance in the living room: salsa, the only dance you need to know. Loosely partnered, my right hand holds his left, my left arm is loose around his waist area, dip-touch forward on right, shift back on left, repeat, then open the grip to face him, and we both are smiling—grinning, really. The music is fat and brassy. We hold onto each other, tight enough to build momentum and pull, snap together, and change direction. There's this thing to figure out: how to keep the steps tight, close enough to whirl, swing open against the one arm on my back, keep at it, and begin to shine. How does dancing with a partner take hold when touch is so complicated? We keep returning to each other like magnets; our bodies calibrate the optimal distance and tone of weight and flesh. Twenty years later, it's called choreography. It is partnering, a lexicon of strategies, feelings, and processes developed and scavenged over time. I don't know if partnering infers meaning, but there is a kind of story-ness; the space between us carries a sense of each of our histories. The silent voice of a gesture is inserted into a sequence of *dream-move-dream* moves, calibrating a landing, the resolve of an action. But back in 1966, it's such a pleasure to wait for the beat to land, to read where the dancing is headed.

In the same year, at the Queensbridge Houses under the Queensboro Bridge: You go down a hallway on the first floor, the 6/8 rhythm of Ghanaian drumming meets you, the door stays open. Nana Yao Opare "Gus" Dinizulu, born in Georgia but living in Queens, traces his lineage back to Ghana. He is a large man who grounds the room as you'd expect. Dinizulu African Dancers, Drummers, and Singers is "the oldest African dance company in America," and its members lead the classes.[3] There's dancing, yes, but also folk milling around, talking and eating in between the fast footwork, arms thrown, lines of folk pounding the floor in "Praise be!" shouts to the drummers. Dinizulu holds *bembés,* ceremonial gatherings from Yoruba religious practice, which generate their own sexual, mystical heat and power through rhythm and time and folk. The drumming goes on for hours, everyone traveling counterclockwise around the large space. The drumming closes my eyes and holds me still in a trance, the flow of dancers dividing and regathering past me; I've been taken. I'm allowed just to be, until I breathe again and I'm back again, in time and flow, with everyone. We own this ground.

1970. Folk dancing on Friday nights at Earl Hall, Columbia University; I'm twenty years old. The line of women and men is resilient: thumbs hooked into their neighbors' belt loops, arms threaded through their partner's, wrists with elbows weighted and loose, feet stamping hard on the bare wood floor. You twist your body a bit to face the line of direction, a taut paper-doll

3 Nana Yao Opare Dinizulu, quoted in "Yao Opare Dinizulu, Troupe Founder, 60," *New York Times*, February 16, 1991.

chain. We rise and fall as a group as the linked volume of us vacuums up the floor. The syncopated footwork sends my body in a chain reaction upward and away. And I own this ground, too!

Once again, I belong to a collective: the Macedonian, Serbian, Balkan dancers; the Greek, Israeli, Scottish bands of folk who dance. I don't know how I found this place, but the door was open; it was hot inside and very sexy. Israeli-born twin brothers, Sabras, play hand drum and violin. They are my age, skinny in black pants and white shirts, sweating—we are all sweating, wet with rhythm; is it a five-, six-, or an eleven-beat measure? I can't tell. The intensity of twenty-somethings eyeing one another, breathing together to an odd-metered beat, the joy, the pounding, all of it is intoxicating.

I love the Black girl folk/salsa/*bembé* dancer in me; I love my knack with foot-work applied to a tricky beat; I love the conglom-erate of motion that is possible, given the choice. Again, choice. Again, where's the tether, what's in the periphery, just out of sight? Each of us is the result of our singular revelations. There is no other job to do, just this.

Timing is becoming essen-tial, naming the rhythm less so. Sound is spatial; action flows in space and story. The range between rhythmic forms—West African, Balkan, dance-class modern, somatic silence, sound scores, North African *bendir,* and Cuban conga beats—shapes how one *might* pay attention if distinctions need to be made. Timing is becoming a *way* of dancing, a rein-terpretation of the pull of sequence and pulse. The conflict of rhythms inside my own body begins to shape gesture; flow becomes overrated. The act of dancing in time and in company feels radiant; it is a new politics that acts like a healing, a joining. The incongruent cultural and political span is part of the pull. Difference is the friction. The *who* of the company you keep when dancing is part of the generative rupture. The span of approaches, of cadence, is packaged in the linked arms, the clan circling the arena. We are kin. We dance.

1978. Context depends on timing, among other things. Certain groups are problematic to define when seen from the outside. In 1978, a reviewer of Alvin Ailey American Dance Theater writes, "Ailey's style... has been seminal...in defining the black dancer's image, an image the next generation copies or rebels against—mostly copies."[4] So: which image shall I choose, assuming there's a choice? Which choice did Raymond Johnson make twenty years earlier? I am most taken by how dancing feels in my body; my Blackness is evident—there is nothing to demonstrate. And who wouldn't want to be a rebel, given the choice? Given that we contain multitudes, the choice is ours in what to manifest. What gets tricky is what's expected from Black dance and Black dancers, and from which corner. Trickier still when allegiance, curiosity, and the market get shuffled together.

St. Mark's Church in-the-Bowery burns almost to the ground six months before the Alvin Ailey review. Months before the fire, Nina Wiener and Dancers (me included) perform at Danspace Project in St. Mark's Church, a work in progress in a space

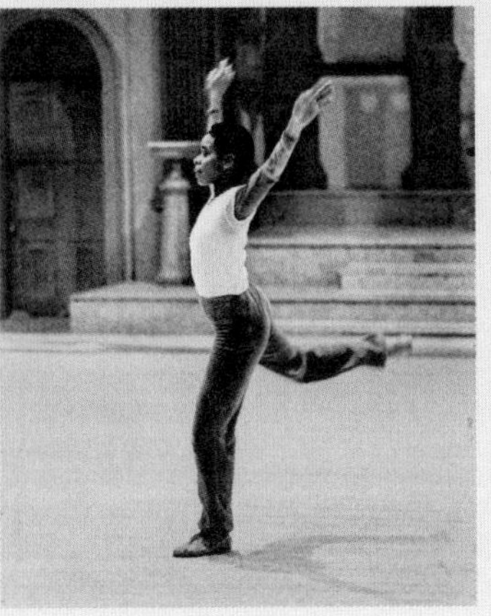
Bebe Miller at St. Mark's Church in-the-Bowery, 1978. Photo by Nathaniel Tileston

that in itself is still in progress. Nina's work presents me with a technical challenge—balance on one leg while completing complicated arm gestures—as well as the more existential issue of what kind of dancing is interesting to do, regardless of the expectations. Where does

4 Deborah Jowitt, "Pearl Remembered to Bring Drummers," *Village Voice*, December 18, 1978.

one show up? When does it matter? Who is watching? Following one's curiosity also means leaving some connections behind, if only to anchor the long end of the tether to where we've come from. One remains oneself.

1982. Ishmael Houston-Jones asks Cynthia Hedstrom, the director of Danspace Project at St. Mark's Church in-the-Bowery, about curating a program that would feature Black choreographers working "outside the Mainstream of Modern Dance."[5] She says yes. In the program notes for the resulting *Parallels*, Houston-Jones goes on to say, "If there is an implicit 'message' to be gotten from this series, it is that this new generation of black artists—who exist in the parallel worlds of Black America and of new dance—is producing work that is richly diverse."[6] True, though, how do you talk about the giddy collision of forms and contents that were suddenly available to each of the artists involved? Blondell Cummings's *Chicken Soup* is my first viewing of her filmic stop-action style of motion, sequencing through hurt and pain and joy. I am slightly mortified by her wire scrub brush actually scrubbing the floor, her wielding of that heavy cast-iron fry pan. My list of what we are *not* supposed to show about Black folk is not far under my skin. When faced with evidence of what free expression looks like, I find it hard to remove the habit of racial judgment, hard to reimagine Blackness in a public space. Ralph Lemon wears a skirt in *Wanda in the Awkward Age,* sharing a concept, keeping clear of meaning. My own piece, *Vespers*, is made of a phrase with variations, danced mostly in silence and to Gregorian chants sung by a dear friend. Much of it is improvised, which feels like I'm cheating whoever is keeping score. I have fallen in love with a way of being by just dancing, and I am relieved not to have to explain how this has come to pass.

5 Ishmael Houston-Jones, "Curatorial Statement," in *Parallels: Danspace Platform 2012* (New York: Danspace Project, 2012), 19.

6 Program notes for *Parallels*, Danspace Project, October 28–30, November 4–6, 1982.

Most of the other works are lost to me, but I remember Ishmael's mother talking about her son while he carries her over his shoulder. (A year or so later/earlier, this same mother's son is dancing, transformed: he has wrapped himself in a fresh goatskin. He has become *creature.* Enthralling, it's another choice I hadn't seen coming.) All of the *Parallels* dances jostle with form in ways that suggest a direction I might try. Their Blackness (our Blackness) and their art making are unmistakable and unassignable, lovely and weird. These particulars seduce me.

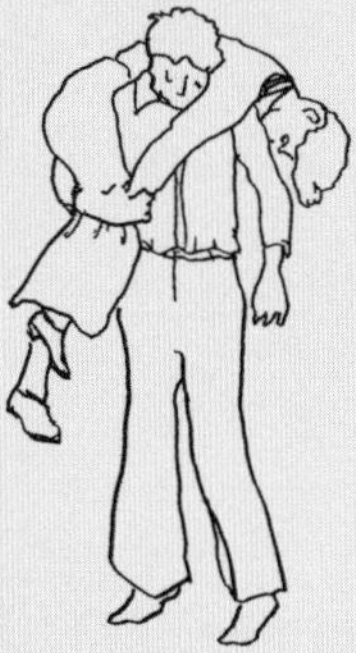

Five years later, Ishmael is invited to bring *Parallels* (now titled *Parallels in Black*) to Europe; Jawole Willa Jo Zollar, the director of the newly formed Urban Dance Women, joins the group. Jawole's piece, *LifeDance...The Fool's Journey*, involves a raw egg. She's wearing boots and a crazy black hat, and she crushes the egg on her chest. We perform in Geneva, London, and Paris—the Josephine Baker Contingent, as dancer Fred Holland calls us—where we're trailed by a police car as we walk down the street. It's hard to gauge the European understanding of the complicated business of race in America. A white audience member in London suggests that Ralph's work is not really Black, not enough. Ralph is surprised and is about to answer when I butt in with a "Who do you think you are?" back talk at the man. I am surprised at myself. Who knows what the man hears of this, as his mind is already made up.

1985. Susan Marshall's work *Arms* is performed at Dance Theater Workshop. Arthur Armijo wraps Susan in an embrace, a takedown that folds her in half again and again. The weighted force is unexpected every time, though I know they've rehearsed this sequence and they both know what's coming. Performing it calls for the perfect combination of care and forceful intention: do no harm, attend to your partner, and agree to whatever emerges. The effort in Arthur's arms is frightening, cradling while forcing her body down; Susan holds her own.

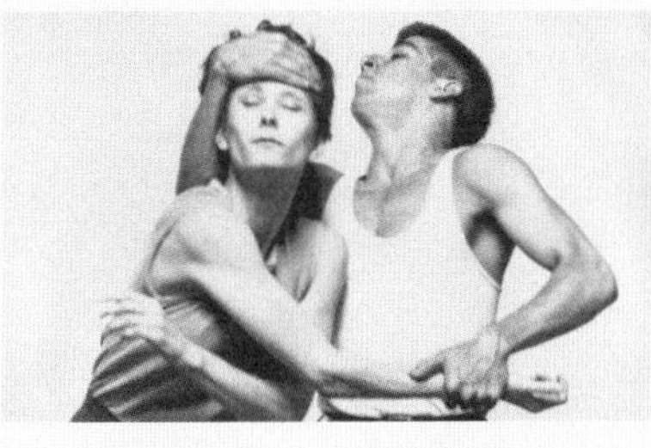

Arthur Armijo and Susan Marshall in Marshall's *Arms*, 1984. Photo by Lois Greenfield

She presses her forehead against his palm while Arthur pulls her wrist to his side, twisted beyond what she might have expected. As I said, Susan holds her own, but her indirect attending-to clinches it for me. And again, the pull-down-takedown, the interrupted timing of the body's recovery from this small assault. Because I know that they are friends and what it takes to shape a moment we can believe, the rehearsal of this action is most intriguing for me. They each draw on a private reserve of tone and *story-ness* to inhabit just for the moment.

Story-ness carries a sense of known history and possible future; linear dance narratives ride on top, secondary to the distilled references that speak to us when we're watching a dance *happen.* Choreography depends on these private decisions to offer up what we've witnessed. The sequence of events, the captured syntax of timing, response, reconsideration, and decision is the driver: do *this* now. The simplicity of Marshall's *Arms*—five minutes long—is still humbling. It changed what I thought dancing could say. It changed how I thought dances could be made. Its insistent, repetitive form seemed an objective, visceral choice between possible outcomes. Choreography calls for curious gatekeepers, and so much depends on what we let into the room.

1986. Ralph Lemon and I are in a studio somewhere, learning something about who we are and how we might dance together. Truth be told, it was Liz Thompson, then the director of Jacob's Pillow, who brought up the idea of a duet, though what we share at this point, besides our Blackness, isn't clear. What would we make? In *Two,* our duet, a man and a woman, well...In the studio, I feel the submerged weight of countless duets between Black men and Black women, called upon to display a particular aspect of domestic rupture.

I don't know what Ralph feels. We don't know each other well at all. I'm blindsided; I take on a role that, really, no one has asked for. Who knew where we would go? Our dancing feels violent, or loving, or instinctive, or driven, given the day. I portray a Black woman, which is not the same as discovering which one I might be. In performance, I feel I am speaking for someone else, though I know exactly what's being said. At the end of *Two,* we stand very close, panting. Ralph bites off a dreadlock just before I turn away. A decade or so later, in *Three*, the film adaptation made by Isaac Julien with Cleo Sylvestre, we continue sniffing our way toward who these people are. At a certain point, there is nothing to decipher; reentry is all.

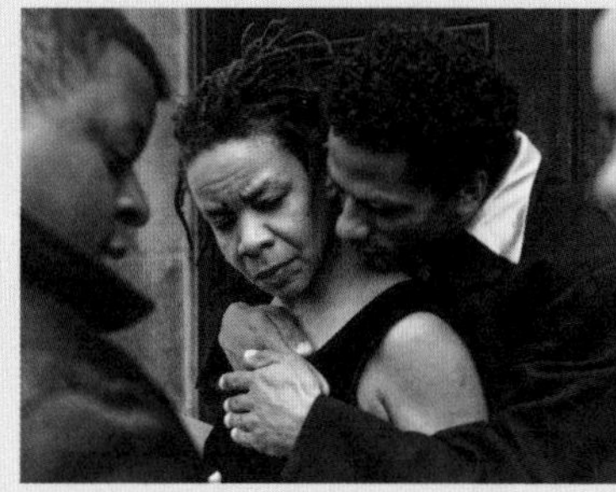

Ralph Lemon and Bebe Miller on set for Isaac Julien's film *Three*, 1999. Photo by Chelsea Lemon Fetzer

Susan and Arthur, and Bebe and Ralph: each duet speaks for itself. Each couple dances through a segment of living before our eyes, solving nothing. I want to place our makings side by side, see the pace of rehearsing, see who thinks of what, see when no one knows what to do next, see what is tossed out, what is called back, and what is never defined.

+++

I spend years dancing, making dances, watching dances. Sniffing out a timing, noting the torque of a body, navigating the politics both in and outside the studio. The lexicon grows. The syntax shifts. What is rendered is a reordering of the old stories, abstracted or literal. One kinetic tone offsets another, the rains are invited, the enemy is conquered, the sun is called. We see her/his/my gesture, the arcing of the side of her/his/my neck toward touch, the improbable posture of arms held at a particular angle of anticipation. My journal notes describe the aimed-for action, the perpendicular relationship, the interrupted vectors of approach. I imagine Ishmael deciding on the goat carcass because he must. I watch Susan decide, with Arthur, how many times she's taken down. I watch Jawole deciding on the egg: yes, she must. We watch Alvin Ailey ask for the next movement based on where the dancers have taken him, where they've been 'buked, where they've been scorned...[7] We feel him lean forward, breathe, sling out his arms, lift his elbows...and watch the moment being captured. The first time is the one to keep; the next is a guess aimed toward all you remember the moment to hold.

7 I am referencing here the gospel hymn "I've Been 'Buked," which accompanies the "Pilgrim of Sorrow" section in Ailey's *Revelations*.

What to choose: *a goatskin*

a garbage-can lid

a raw egg

your mother over your shoulder

a 6/8 beat, or none

a dream move

a partner

one story

What is available:
everything.

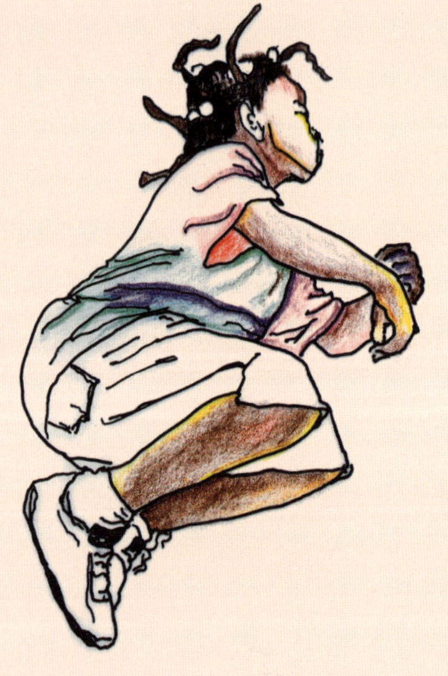

Once upon one kinda time,
I wanted to be the Vietnamese Irish
Maria Tallchief when I grew up.
I didn't have the body.

For the record, I can write actual sentences. *Do* academia. I've taught dance history and championed, demanded, and celebrated the retirement of Dance in the Twentieth Century as the catchall. Renamed it Global, acknowledged the hubris of a scope like the Whole Planet while talking down panic at the dissolving ego of the dance canon, and pondered with graduate students on the entrapment of linear time along with the "human contradiction"[1] of insisting on certain superiorities and authorities as dominant in historical representation. I've wrangled. I've wrestled. But I am NOT a historian or a herstorian or a nonbinarian representative of any kind of This Was or Was Not.

I'm just here with my octo-self . . . tentacular,[2] decentral, a-linear, fluid AF . . . like a life.

This is gunna be salty. This is gunna be hot and wet and full o' sweat.
And tears.
And years.
And years.
And years.
No years.
Fuck chronos.
Fuck front to back.
Fuck line, fuck all noncyclical time.

1 In Octavia Butler's *Xenogenesis* trilogy (aka *Lilith's Brood*), the "human contradiction" refers to the unfortunate and lethal combination of high intelligence and hierarchical thinking.

2 Thank you, Donna J. Haraway, for *Staying with the Trouble: Making Kin in the Chthulucene* (Durham, NC: Duke University Press, 2016).

This I know
we will reap cuz, damn, we did sow,
sowed and growed, like the whole
dang dia-spora.
so . . .
hold up . . . look down . . . 3, 2, 1 . . .
hair toss . . .
ok go . . .

Time: The Beginning . . . Or? . . .
A beginning?
Place: Việt Nam

Serpent lord and bird goddess
A dragon to a fairy
The Sea to the Sky[3]
One hundred eggs bore one hundred babes
Fifty stayed high
Fifty dropped low
And that was how it'd go

In the beginning, it was a mystical duet
then a large group work filled with
level changes,
sites
and sex
and sexes
and exits and exes

A supernatural selection

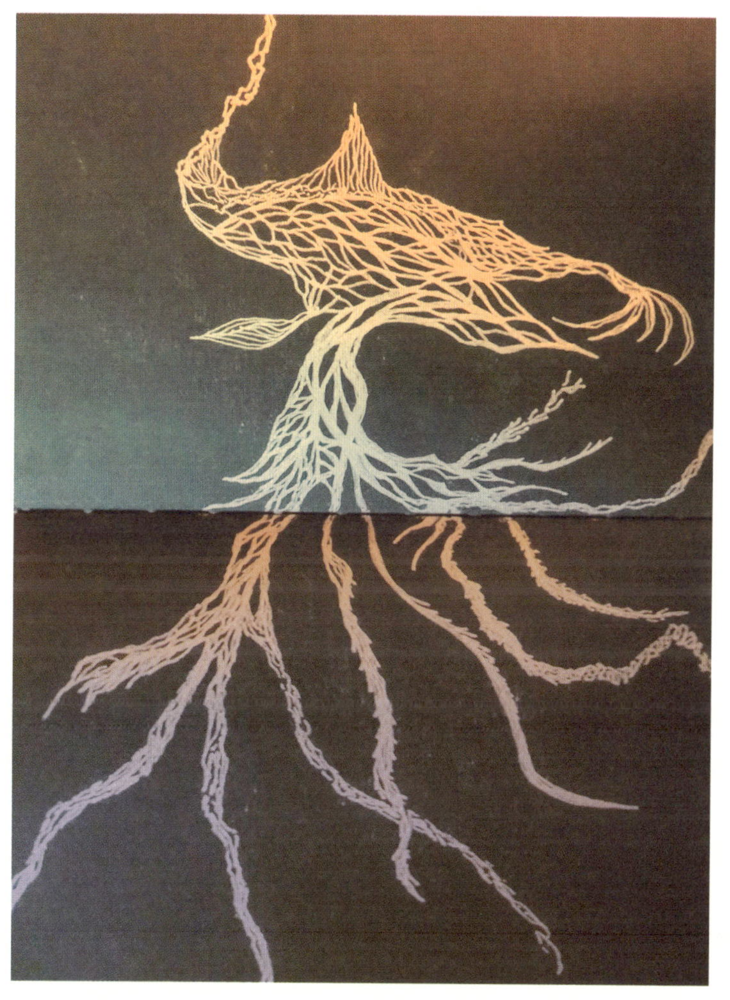

3 Vietnamese origin myth.

Time (travel)

We take our time. We keep time.
We waste time. We step out of time.

1. Place yourself in a memory.
   Bring it back fully, in as many senses as you can. Remember yourself in that memory.
2. Project yourself into a plan for the future. Fill out the fantasy fully. Envision yourself in this future.
3. Switch places. The memory is a plan; the plan is a past. Let it become far in the past.

How does it change your nervous system
to reconfigure lines into cycles?[4]

Who took the music away from the dance?
Can I have it back now, please,
ye ol' Pure Dance?

There are dancers engraved on Đông Sơn drums from 600 BCE. That is 2,621 years ago…so…yeah… *Let Me Hear Ya Say Bass.*[5]

So, like I said, not a historian nor an archaeologist, a once-upon-a-time anthro major at best, so that creation myth…yeah, it's a bit Chinese-y, it doesn't get the Kingdom of Champa or the Cham people who found their way to central and southern Việt Nam via the sea. It doesn't carry Lady Po Nagar, who descended from the mountains, floated to China on sandalwood, had a couple of kids with the crown prince, fled home by flinging her sandalwood into the ocean, disappearing with the kids and reappearing on the beaches of Nha Trang. I mean, the bit where she turns the Chinese prince and his fleet into stone when they try to follow her is e.v.e.r.y.thing. Our own Medusa, with Southeast Asian serpent worship (Naga/Nagi) and reclaimed survivor tales, y'all…I receive the Mother Lode's download. Light that Nag Champa, get to praying![6]

Who took me dance away from me music? Can I go home again, please?

I spora, you spora, we all spora for the Dia Spora.

English speakers call the thousand-year-old form Chèo theater, but it's dance, but it's musical theater, but it's political, but it's popular. Hát Chèo is a cultural treasure; it was started by a royal dancer (Mrs.) Phạm Thị Trân during the House of Đinh, Việt Nam's first independent dynasty, but it's folk now cuz it was exiled by House of Lê Duy monarch Lê Thánh Tông, emperor of Đại Việt from 1460 to 1497. He wanted more poets in the court. So it became common, a commoner's form. I don't do it, never did, but it's in my bones to be theatrical, so I claim descendancy.

4 Grown from a Camae Ayewa (Moor Mother) and Rasheedah Phillips (Black Quantum Futurism) exercise in time travel.

5 Beat Mafia, "Let Me Hear Ya Say Bass," 1995.

6 Thank you, j. bouey, for helping to return my recovering Catholic sense to the idea of prayer as an intentional orientation of energy.

The younger thirteenth-century Tuồng is defined as opera, but it's Chinese opera, but it's the Vietnamese version of Chinese opera, so it's chock-full o' gender-bender fancy dancy, but it's an imperial gift, a colonizer's form. Or no, maybe it's about a captured Mongol, Lý Nguyễn Cát, who was forced to teach the royals a form that persisted in high popularity until the last dynasty, when the House of Nguyễn abdicated after World War II, following French and Japanese occupation. I absolutely identify with the drag and the drums, with the clash of military tales, romantic conquest, and a LOT of makeup. My trans and nonbinary offspring are the blossoms of these gender- and genre-fluid forms, seeded into being before communist and capitalist codification of co-ed-ification congealed.

A quick history of my body inside Asian forms: Tai Chi Sword for H. T. Chen and Dancers in lec dem after lec dem; Peking Opera Troupe No. 1 and *M. Butterfly* choreographer, Jamie H. J. Guan, and I doing two-person Chinese opera versions of the Monkey King (Jamie = Monkey King, me = all of heaven and earth) all over the northeastern and midwestern United States; ribbon dancing kokken in Berkeley Repertory Theater's *Dragonwings* in Seattle, Atlanta, and Syracuse; Korean mask dancing at the Seoul Institute of the Arts during my first La MaMa Great Jones Rep tour in 1997; monkey dances in the dirt courtyard of Sovanna Phum in Phnom Penh during one of several Dance Theater Workshop residencies in Southeast Asia; tai chi and qigong in Oakland's Chinatown with the old ladies; yoga and a yoga honeymoon and a yoga family trip at the Sivananda Ashram on Paradise Island and yoga at every fucking gym everywhere; ten silent days of Vipassana in Shelburne Falls, Massachusetts; advanced brown belt in Seido karate with Kaicho Tadashi Nakamura;

performing butoh in Yokohama and Tokyo with Kazuo and Yoshito Ohno; a bit o' tae kwon do and maybe it was wushu with the Asian stunt team for *Warrior.*

How far out must we go in order to earn a return to the source?

There is no quick history of all I witnessed, watched, or wrote about in Cambodia, Hong Kong, India, Japan, Laos, New York, Taiwan, Thailand, and Việt Nam for the *Dance Insider* or *Culturebot* or the two different New York Dance and Performance Awards committees I cochaired or the Congress on Research in Dance, Movement Research, Dance Theater Workshop, the Field, and DANCE NOW boards and arts councils I sat on. *All you touch and all you see is all your life will ever be...*[7] There is no way back to a wayback before the waybackmachine could archive the website of Dance Theater Workshop's multiyear *Mekong Project,* which I codeveloped, conducted research for, and facilitated residencies for in Southeast Asia and New York for Mekong Delta and American diasporic artists. That last gig in Hong Kong with Julian Barnett, Abby Chan, Christopher Morgan, and Becky Jung (rest with the ancestors you found soon after that project) required Perry Yung to run around the city with #1 packed on his back and #2 strapped to his chest. Old Chinese women yelling, *Where's the mother???* all over Kowloon. After that, we just had to put down the root system and tune into the mycelium, ease off the sporing, and forget that things are quite different somewhere and somewhen else.

7 Pink Floyd, "Breathe (In the Air)," 1973.

Is history about the past?
Is history about the passed?

At this moment, in this writing, I sit in grief. I recognize that someone's departure from the planet opens new space for connection and appreciation in some kind of collective remembering but makes the absence of access to a quiet, resilient source acute. Nai-Ni Chen, you held that Asian immigrant culture was American culture. 谢谢. Corky Lee, our photographer laureate of Asian America and that guy who will do your postcards for your upcoming Dance Theater Workshop show cheap, too soon, too soon. Jun Maeda-san, I still cut cans into ribbons in the way you showed Jet Yung and me when we'd sit with you every Tuesday after school in your La MaMa basement workshop as you wove the strands into a phoenix, into "artistic" things. Anna's dad, Edwina Cummings, bell hooks, Nicole's mom, Desmond Tutu. There's one day left in this Julian calendar. Has the quota been filled yet?

Six months later or last week, Erik Ehn, playwright and former CalArts dean, Brown MFA director turned theologist, said on a Great Jones Rep Zoom reading of his latest plays: *Together, we make a wheel, and so we turn and turn and turn and re-turn.*

I can hear Robin Wall Kimmerer, in that gentle and tender voice, reminding me to remember:

> *A species and a culture that treat the natural world with respect and reciprocity will surely pass on genes to ensuing generations with a higher frequency than the people who destroy it. The stories we choose to shape our behaviors have adaptive consequences.*[8]

How far back do we go to know who we are? Remember. Join the remembering.

Feel your energy rooting into the ground below you. Sense yourself spreading the roots of you. Rub your belly for a minute. Take a deep breath. Fill out a picture of your closest ancestor in your mind. Invite them to entangle their roots with yours. Thank them for offering the foundation on which you grow the new world.[9]

When is the beginning of a thing? When did we dance together first, Sasa? Our duets in Yoshito Ohno's butoh classes in Yokohama were the first conscious dances I danced with you. And there was Kazuo Ohno still dancing, rolling into the studio and passionately gesturing whenever Elvis's "How Great Thou Art" would play. Perry Yung and I were welcomed to his ninety-fourth birthday because La MaMa—Ellen Stewart—presented him first in the United States. And so we were family. Thanks, MaMa.

Bruce Lee said, *Notice that the stiffest tree is most easily cracked, while the bamboo or willow survives by bending with the wind.*[10]

We bred for change; we bred us-selves for adaptability, agility, resilience, to grow like weeds, like bamboo, to propagate in rhizomatic glory.

Dance is my weed. Six months ago, Erik Ehn said on a (different) La MaMa Great Jones Rep Zoom call: *Theater is a refugee art form.* But he don't know what dance has to do. Always. So often in flight, leaping to avoid unfriendly ground. Or digging. It has to sink,

8 Robin Wall Kimmerer, *Braiding Sweetgrass: Indigenous Wisdom, Scientific Knowledge and the Teachings of Plants* (Minneapolis: Milkweed Editions, 2013), 30.

9 maura nguyễn donahue, "Education," in *Justice. Transformation. Education: Reimagining the Dance Ecology*, ed. Candace Zachery (New York: Dance/NYC Symposium, 2021), 70; https://www.dance.nyc/uploads/untitled%20folder/DanceNYC-Symp2021-Program-210315B.pdf.

10 Bruce Lee, *Artist of Life* (Boston: Tuttle, 1999), 32.

root, and forage…seek nutrient-rich soil or toil on rocky outcrops like a bristlecone. Hoping to last past the first couple of rough, arid years and then outlast the Roman Empire. Dance is a refuge, but dancers are increasingly the refugees.

Who took the people away from the dance? Can they please come home now?

Marc Morozumi! Remember how, as emerging artists, we documented everyone's cuts and bruises after our Vietnamese refugee piece at Bates Dance Festival? Paul Matteson was so proud of his. *Twenty-one-year spill*, a diasporic ooze with all the dancers falling down the side of that hill. Over those rocks. Winding our web of ropes around all the trees. So many tendrils running into the open field and lashed back. Remember how Nia Love was the only person supportive of our *Exotic Dancers* piece? Remember how we shared a house with Contraband and laughed at how one of them always cried after our yoga class? RIP Kathleen Hermesdorf. Do you remember when we were on tour in Massachusetts and you woke me in the middle of the night because you'd gotten crabs after apartment-sitting for a certain former ___ dancer, now ___ professor? Do you remember when we did that project with the Vietnamese youth in Springfield, Massachusetts, went to Bates, did a shitload of contact improvisation, came back to New York and continued our exotic dancers' exploration by working in Times Square (my club was definitely more fun than yours), and finally realized I didn't have dandruff but had probably given lice to a shit ton of the denizens of Runway 69? The 1900s were seriously a ratchet time.

Peggy Cheng, Nancy Ellis, SanSan Kwan, and Brian Nishii, remember that time I thought maybe Maura Nguyễn Donohue/InMixedCompany could be the Asian American Contraband, but with taiko drums? Rick Ebihara, MiRi Park, Wayland Quintero, and Perry Yung, remember how I just gave the band job over to you all for *Lotus Blossom Itch* and *Strictly a Female Female*? Peggy, do you remember Keely Garfield taking you for a walk around Performance Space 122 on a leash for *Rip It Open*? Keely doesn't know this, but I wanted to be the AAPI Keely when I grew up. I didn't have the charm.

Out on a limb, let's get back to the bristlecone seedling. If our dance lasts the first couple of years, we might end up among the longest-living organisms on the planet. There's a tree that's twice as old as the Bronze Age Vietnamese drum somewhere out there. Let's remember all the dances from before the People. The spores on the wind, fantastic in flight.

Let's start in the ground, let's start with rooting our feet and sinking our weight. Let's *bond with the earth*; let's *graze*. Let's remember Nancy Stark Smith for taking us down into the soil with her Underscore improvisational scores. Remember her giggles during Triangle Arts sharings with artists from Indonesia, Japan, and the United States at the Bates Dance Festival? Let's breathe and touch something. Let's recognize that she left the planet right at a moment when touch had become fugitive and contact was criminal.

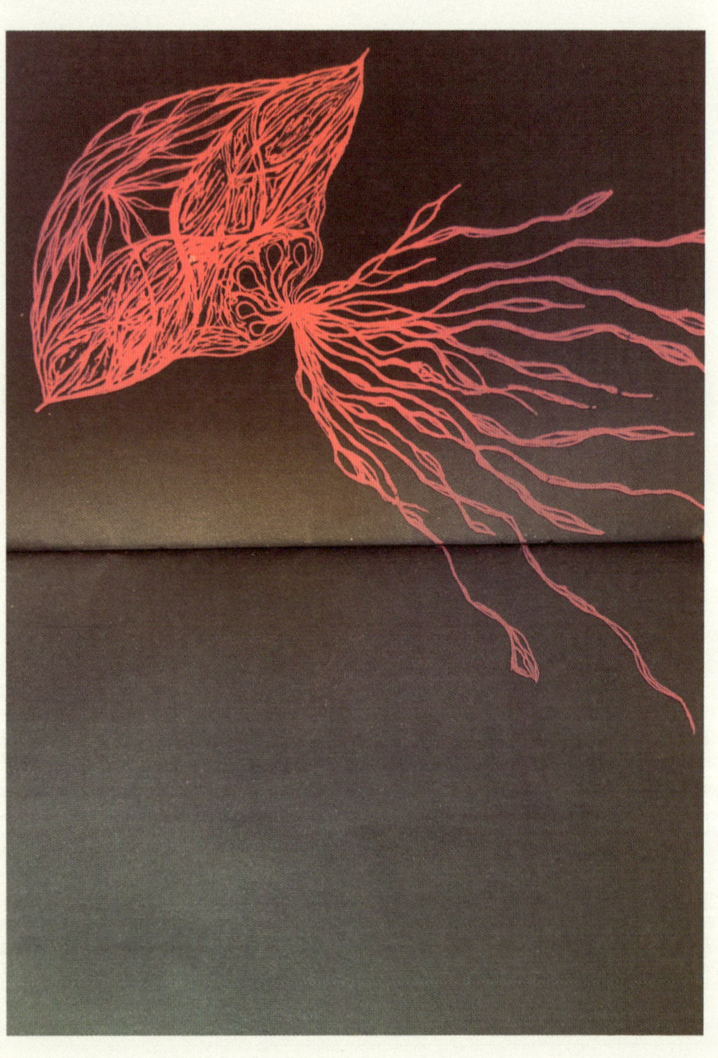

Dance is a cephalopod
so let's start in the sea,
slippery,
unruly in captivity,
and
tentacular.

Evolve
and
colonize
land
like
the first fungi.

Dance is a weed. So let's start in the ground; let's find the mycorrhizal networks, let's find the Mother Tree, and let's nourish each other in the dark, dank unknown.[11] Let's start with the rhythms that found their way from my heart to yours, for that bump, for the current and the currency of our blood, the pulse and the thrum.

Let's start in the ground, let's start with the vibration that wends its way from origin blossom to *so full of myself that my cup runneth over…*[12] Let's remove the rubber sole, feel the dirt under our toes, let's press in and shift slightly, bend our knees, elbows, and wrists, open our eyes, raise our fingers, shift out the hips, and begin a classical Khmer dance like we are one of the remaining 10 percent after Pol Pot tried to kill everyone. Let's remember when a royal dance became resistance in the refugee camps of Thailand, when it was gifted to Sophiline Cheam Shapiro like a seed carried through an apocalypse, when a nation considered it among its

11 Suzanne Simard, *Finding the Mother Tree: Discovering the Wisdom of the Forest* (New York: Knopf, 2021).

12 Creatrx, "Sunday," 2021.

priorities to rebuild the arts in the blood-soaked wake of the Khmer Rouge. When a princess made it illegal to change the apsaras and Sophi became a renegade.

Let's start in the ground; I'll meet you in the mud. In the muddy waters of the Mekong River Delta. In the Proto-Austroasiatics,[13] the southern parts, in the Proto-Mon–Khmer, in the times before we spoke what is spoken and just danced what sometimes is still dancin'. Let's *wade in the water/Remember how we used to wade in the water/Now we twerk in the water, twerk, twerk in the water/This is a freedom dance/Gon' assume the stance/Shake it like you got one chance/To let the rain free, And set the pain free, Can't let'em train we/Respectability, nah that ain't me/It never made us free/Or help plant our seeds/Or help grow our trees/I be who I be/So I honor that sacred racthetry . . .*[14]

Let's sing up our own song of becoming and becoming and becoming. Let's create the vibrations beyond glottal stops or pitch-perfect specifics in meaning. Let's jump from Cham to Chad peoples, from Iron Age Southeast Asia to the end of the Second French Colonial Empire. From the Indigenous to the independent. Let's find ourselves across aspirations and fundamental frequencies, and let us not separate our songs from our dances; let us remember to be distinctive in our differences and fertile foreigners in our storytelling. Let's tune out. Let's unparent ourselves from our pasts; let's generate a hyper-popped-out screech fest of ancient alien wondrousness; let's tell the hidden tales, reinscribe the walls with bits of our bodies that seeped out, oozed from every orifice; let's give the larynx and the patella to the cause of becoming real.

Take the larynx.
Take the language.
Take the lungs and the lilt
of tonal dialects.
I cannot write my way into the
dances I've danced.

The edge of the words are the edges of a world forming, alpha terra bite down and drown in absentia in what is unsaid, what dissolves into predictable transmission when those structures can't surround us. When what it is to tell you is not the same as to convey, when what must be conveyed cannot be communicated, when the metamorphosis of meaning into the materiality of language butchers the great beauty of us. Where you say, *you will tell me*, but I tell you as Actaeon told his hounds not to slay him, transfigured from an apex predator to the bottom of the chain. What I say is not what I mean, what I tell is underneath the saying, where unfathomable is the way down to the bottom of this thing we are trying to do to this big to-do to do something without quantity without quality without frivolity without within and without comprehending without defining as we defy bounds of saying things, say what?

I don't wanna write the thing because the thing is the thing and the words are not the thing and the righting the words is not the thing and it's just writing.

I cannot say to anyone what I want to matter, to become matter to form to fill to follow a whim to a thought to a want to a do. What do I listen to? Or who.

13 The ancestral language of mainland Southeast Asia.

14 Creatrx, "Baptism," 2018.

Digging below the tongue, unclipping a voice from the orator, there isn't any way I will not end up a traitor to every other pathway possible that I might have said. How do I answer so that the choosing is not about losing? Once said, once read if beyond the spaciousness in my head, there will be only the linear, the direct, and the dead dead dead end of language and fixed forms and a focus on clarity and arTiCulAtion and sense and sensibility.

If I could tell you in words, I wouldn't
need so badly to dance. it. out.

What is time-based art when one has
grandmothered to the great unity,
god-moleculed to the source?

The point of the thing isn't the thing itself.
It is nothing.
It is the making of the thing that is the
thing, dig?
No, seriously... I meant dig.
Plant the seedling as if you were Octavia
Butler's heroine in *Parable of the Sower*.

A thing is a known entity.
The making is the world of unknowing.
The cloud of possibility.
Alive
Changing
Eternal

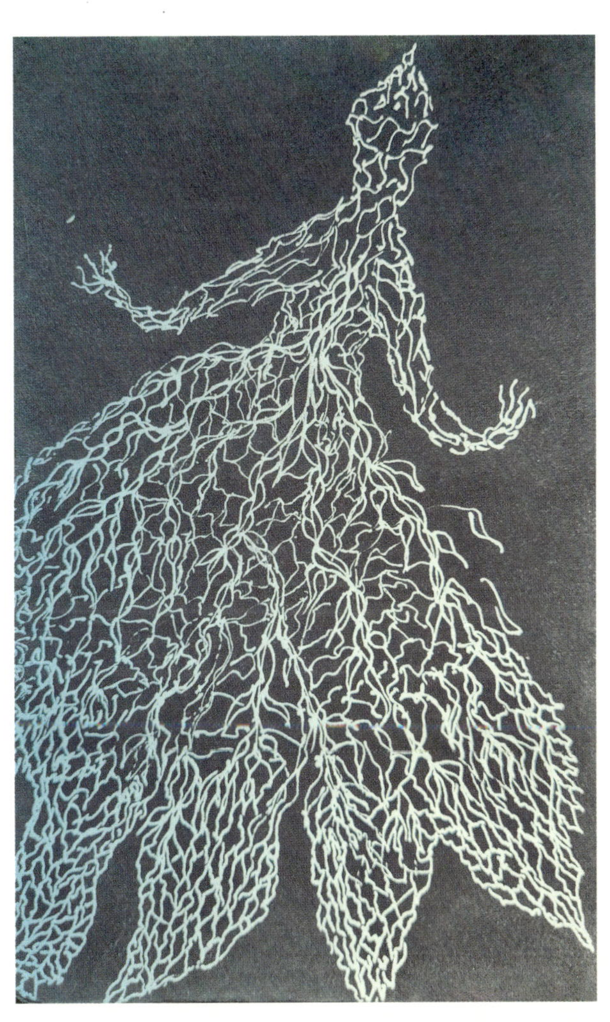

Here is a thing,
a thing I made for you.
But it is nothing.
No thing of value.

It is the time.
The feeling of my hand upon it.
Spray-on concrete, my aching wrist.

Where was it that this was?
It is not here, and it is not now.

I owe you nothing.
I be myself and I ain't fronting, eh,
nah, nah, nah.[15]

'Cept there are histories that I want learned, to blast the passed over to the stratosphere of learned halls, to make us, the Othered bodies, material, meaningful, mattering. But I owe us a shift into something gentle and joyful in this thick and fevered present, so I will say it simply:

I want you to stop teaching like
Euro-concert dance deserves
pride of place.
Oh, and maybe…just quit it with
the hierarchy of the body?

I want the dances we've danced since before spoken and written language to raise the spirits again. I want the sacrifice and the shaman and the Scheherazadian battle to break through to dawn again and again through a millennium of conjurings.

I want the dance at the fire to live as powerfully as that of the court but not in that, like, y'kno, co-opted, fukkin, 475-plus-140-dollar vehicle-pass-Burning-Man kinda campfire dance kinda way, ri-y-t? I wanna know what a real campfire, *it's a bonfire, turn the lights out…*[16] Harvest dance was like…I wanna dance in the real *Rite of Spring*. I mean…all-night sojourns and plenty o' chemical enhancement have been pursued, but my fire-escape tomatoes do not look as good as Sydnie Mosley's, y'kno'what I'm sayin'. It's like I can *n-ts-n-ts-n-ts-n-ts-n-ts-n-ts-n-ts-n-ts* pound and pulse all night, but then how did my garden grow? Not so…not so much. Because no one taught me the principles of the Honorable Harvest.[17] I have taken the first and the last without asking, more than I needed, even if I do share.

Remember that scene in Hayao Miyazaki's *My Neighbor Totoro* where the children and the sprites dance around the acorns and collectively grow them into a massive camphor tree? That's my dance. Growing bounty through intentional sweat in concerted effort in community. It's the making movement meaningful through conscious attenuation to something outside our single-entity status. It's the god trees of Shinto. It's the animism of EVERY single THING. It's the rooting. It's the barefooted. It's the earth and the Earth.

15 Seinabo Sey, "I Owe You Nothing," 2018.
16 Childish Gambino, "Bonfire," 2011.
17 As detailed in Kimmerer's *Braiding Sweetgrass*.

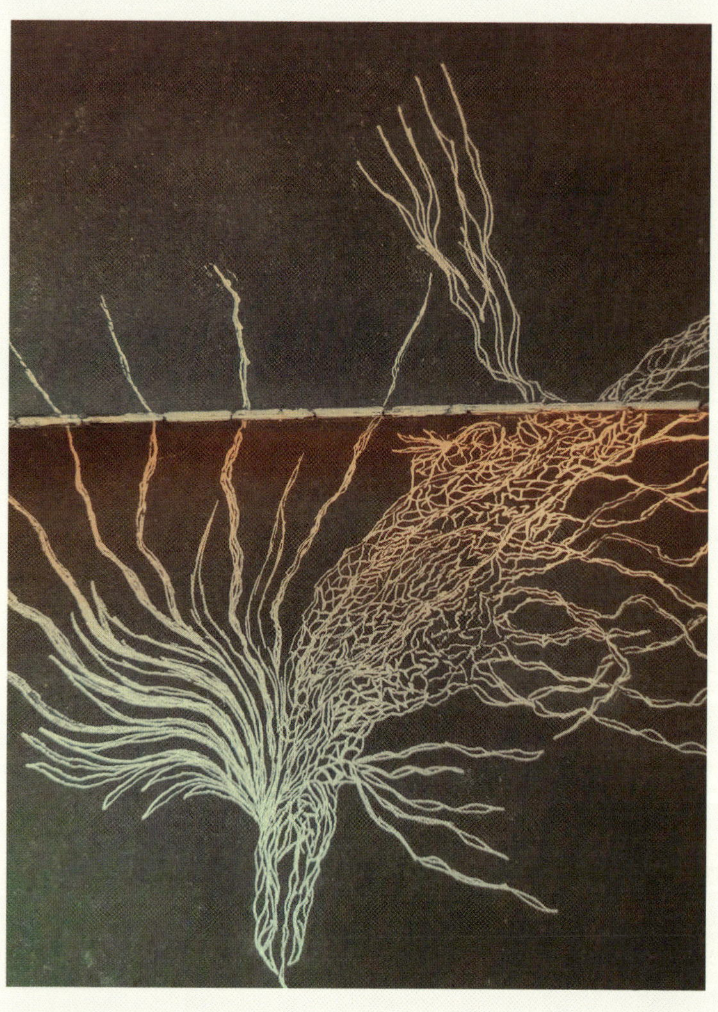

It's as sweet as a Studio Ghibli countryside and as hot and dangerous as a Hanatarashi show.[18] It's coming together to energetically connect into a live circuit at the edges of life and death. It's smashing a bulldozer through the wall as choreo. It's the motherfucking mosh pit at a Prison Religion show with False Prophet screaming from *O FUCC I'M ON THE WRONG PLANET.* It's Reagan Holiday smacking a contact microphone on her ass at Market Hotel while we all hollah.

It's Arca at the Shed. Dragon.
Demon. Deity. @arca1000000 as
a mythical force alighted and lit.

Magical journeys through psychokinetic
raptures and a voluminous luminous.

To have been welcomed into her fold
was an ascendancy of the highest
order and sublimest disorder.

Devoted witnessing was a luscious
intoxicant as we glimpsed an
eternal present.

After college, I thought maybe
I'd be the next Elizabeth Roxas
or Dana Hash and be the
Asian chick in Ailey.
I still didn't have the body.

18 Hanatarashi was infamous for dangerous noise-band shows, including one with a bulldozer that destroyed the back wall of the venue; see https://medium.com/music-voices/how-a-bulldozer-became-a-musical-instrument-67b71c1be48 and http://www5a.biglobe.ne.jp/~gin/rock/japan/hanatarasi/hanatarashi2.html.

In the way back when of experienced lifelines,
I spun you around at Peggy Cheng's wedding, Sasa.
Back then, you'd wear a dress without abolition
or irony. Before T time. But who was the first human
to do such a thing with their offspring? Who shared
the first conscious extraneous gesture on the planet?
What conditions needed to exist for Homo sapiens
to relax into delight with one another? Was it really a
Stanley Kubrick *Space Odyssey* violent celebration
of ape smashing bone onto skull? I know we dance at
the kill, at the touchdown, on the graves of our enemies...
but from this distance, I see into the moment when
dance was the first instance of human play...before
being formalized into ritual; into social; into time, space,
effort; into us/do and them/watch; into I move, you
touch; into Darwinian sexual-selection practices.

I think distance is part of our
cosmic scale,
i said.
Separation is a necessary aspect of...
Togetherness is not the opposite
of separation,
u said...
OK, but,
i said.

You expand and draw me from such a
great distance that my reach will grow.
It's at this distance that we'll fashion
wild new kinespheres.

Scale is the thing to learn from you.
Massive. Magical gestures that strike
at the scope of the normal. In your enormity,
I am blinded.

I see you enormous against the scale
of the world.

I become more obscure, maybe with
you, I can build beyond my small planet
into your void.

At this distance, I draw complex blueprints
for future vessels.
When you are near, there are none.
There is no need to build, to reach,
to grow.

At this distance, I plot courses, plan routes,
survey new territories, recall and anticipate
the travels.

At this distance,
everything is…
is…
available.

Stay. Away.

I need to...*ramble on, sing my song... find my girl...on my way...now's the time, the time is now.*[19]

A colleague at Hunter College and an actual anthropologist, Michael Steiper, sent me an article about humans, symmetry, dance, and mating. I wondered if this is what real contemporary anthropologists do. My 1900s women's-college version of an anthro major meant deconstructing the excessive white cis male arrogance of androcentric anthro while doing past-life regressions, reading Starhawk, studying the anthropology of menstruation with Frédérique Apffel-Marglin, who'd done her fieldwork among the temple dancers of Shree Jagannath, and dancing the dances of the Caribbean with Yvonne Daniel.

Dance is believed to be important in the courtship of a variety of species, including humans, but nothing is known about what dance reveals about the underlying phenotypic—or genotypic—quality of the dancer. One measure of quality in evolutionary studies is the degree of bodily symmetry (fluctuating asymmetry, or FA), because it measures developmental stability. Does dance quality reveal FA to the observer, and is the effect stronger for male dancers than female?[20]

Did I breed more symmetrical bodies than my own out of mating with a more symmetrical body than my own?...I mean...if not for Muna Tseng's *The Pink* at La MaMa and Ellen Stewart in my parents' backyard in Rhode Island in the last days of Y2K, ringing her bell for our backyard wedding, Perry Yung, you and I wouldn't have been singing her coffin out of St. Patrick's Cathedral, tears streaming, the final song of Andrei

Șerban and Elizabeth Swados's *The Trojan Women* resonating, holding Sasa and Jet's little hands. She had me share a room with her on my first Great Jones Repertory tour. She did. not. know. me. but she brought me to South Korea to play Helen of Troy anyway, and I clawed my way back to play her again twenty-five-plus years later. So, yeah. Arrogant, motherfucking, sex-positive bitches. All the shes be in mes. And a couple of Athenas. Why just be hawt when you can be hawt and smawt? But the point is, Ellen Stewart showed me how to be in the world...trust the instinct, give people a chance, and don't let the bastards or the fancy people bring you down, honey.

Every now and then, MFA Darvejon Jones says, *I forgot you a fighter,* and I laugh, but in my post-fifty-me search, I float in Paul Bowman's discursive constellation of martial arts in pop-culture media.[21] Back in undergrad, a drummer for Yvonne Daniel's Monday night Caribbean class asked why I didn't study my own culture's dances: *Why do you wanna only dance Black ways?* At the time, I thought, *'Cuz we don't have dope drums... and everything is supposed to be pretty.* But I took Gemze de Lappe's Duncan class too—that was yt peepl, right? But I heard him. I wont looking. I spent a lot of time asking my form to inhabit forms that excited me, so it was Peking Opera–ish shows with the most fabulous ornamental battles of celestial camp and animal drag. Friends, if you've never seen Leslie Cheung (rest in true peace) in Chen Kaige's *Farewell My Concubine,* you can't begin to imagine the sublime and chaotic twentieth-century Asian queering of desire that is set within the framework of a performance form that uses stylized combat and symbolic gestures for storytelling as much as speech and song and prioritizes the beauty of their movement to assess a performer's skill.

19 Led Zeppelin, "Ramble On," 1969.

20 William M. Brown et al., "Dance Reveals Symmetry Especially in Young Men," *Nature* 438, no. 7071 (December 22, 2005): 1,148–50.

21 Paul Bowman, *The Invention of Martial Arts: Popular Culture between Asia and America* (Oxford, UK: Oxford University Press, 2021).

But there is also the dance of a kata 型 or 形, which literally means "form." Last century, in the BC (before children), there was a shelf full of trophies for kata competitions during my years of training in Seido karate (hello, Billy Macagnone, hello, Rhetta Aleong). Kata is a storytelling form. It performs a slow-motion fight where viewers see only the soloist lunging, turning, kicking, balancing, punching, and blocking an imaginary partner. It is set choreography that asks the practitioner to attenuate and engage performance practices of breath, dynamic shift, tempo alterations, weight shift, and intentional focus. If the now had been the then, I coulda been a media contender. Coulda/shoulda/woulda… There was no US context back then… It was for Michelle Yeoh and Maggie Cheung and Anita Mui to *Heroic Trio*. There wasn't even a Lucy Liu yet, just Anna May Wong and that "Ancient Chinese Secret" laundry commercial to strive for, right, eugene the poogene? I settled for doing katas naked with words like *bitch, cunt,* and *whore* written on me while Ani DiFranco's "I'm No Heroine" lyrics were projected on me. In Bowman's discursive constellation, I was a hot mess of a star.

Dance is believed to be important in the courtship of a variety of species, including humans.

The best pay I ever got as a professional dancer was stripping in Times Square. I'd already been naked all over downtown—why not get paid for a change, right? I funded my Dance Theater Workshop season that way.

A body is a Body only if it transforms the rules of existence.[22]

22 @vvxxii, Instagram post, April 23, 2019.

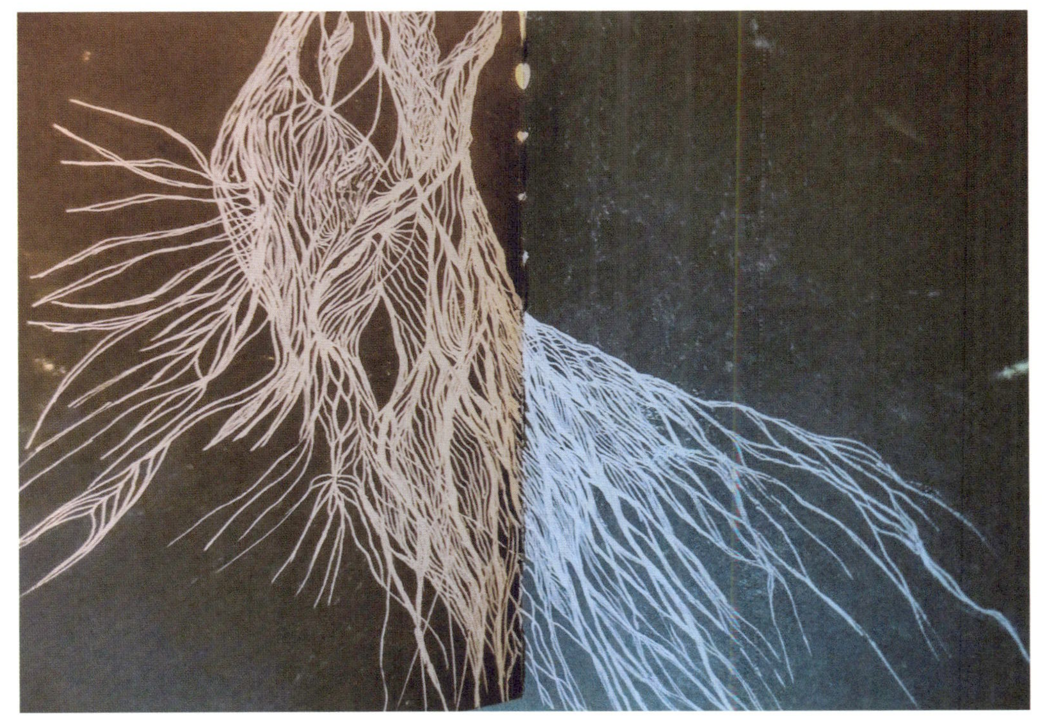

If I map myself crown to toe, seeking the living archive of this vessel, would the scars, the cellulite, the swelling, the pigmentations, stretch marks, tattoos, piercings, asymmetry, amassed mass tell you my history? Does my naming a few names tell you our history? If I were to invoke the as-yet-unnamed legacies, conscious or unconscious *at the time*, of luciana achugar, Elizabeth Alexander, Vanessa Anspaugh, Aretha Aoki, Antonin Artaud, Pina Bausch, Charlotte Brathwaite, adrienne maree brown, Ivica Buljan, Donald Byrd, Pema Chödrön, Ping Chong, Thomas Ciufo, Jessica Colotti, Seán Curran, Kirsten Davis, Gilles Deleuze, Joan Didion, Kristina Dobosz, Bernard G. Donohue Jr., Eirene Donohue, Mai Donohue, David Dorfman, Timothy Edwards, Doug Elkins, devynn emory, Karen Finley, Miguel Gutierrez, Thích Nhất Hạnh, Donna Haraway, Joy Harjo, Keith Hennessy, Pat Hoffbauer, bell hooks, Emily Johnson, Sankai Juku, Sam Kim, Shigeko Kubota, Ralph Lemon, Clarice Lispector, Audre Lorde, Marshall McLuhan, Bebe Miller, Motus, Seta Morton, Graziella Murdocca, Hung Nguyễn, Jennifer Nugent, Mary Oliver, Yoko Ono, Eiko Otake, iele paloumpis, Nicky Paraiso, Robin Prichard, Antonio Ramos, Gilbert Reyes, Dwight Rhoden, Dan Safer, george emilio sanchez, Andrei Șerban, Vicky Shick, Rosy Simas, Annie Sprinkle, Gertrude Stein, Eddie Taketa, lê thị diễm thúy, Roberta Uno, Zisan Urgulu, Reggie Wilson, Kevin Wynn, Yasuko Yokoshi, and Mia Yoo, would I have built a representational constellation of nourishment and formation? Where do I situate Cassie Peterson? What about the beloved, inspirational editors of this collection? To quantify my ineffable experience of artistic influence is to land like the apple in a Newtonian world when I fluctuate into quantum and metaphysical realms. All this material is immaterial.

The struggle with writing a dance history is a struggle with time. What if, somewhere in between Oliver Burkeman's *Four Thousand Weeks: Time Management for Mortals* and Elisabeth Tova Bailey's *The Sound of a Wild Snail Eating*, we let the meaningful progression to a (hopefully) peaceful departure bring us to ourselves as time, not in time, not against time, not out of time.[23] Not a Walter Benjamin reading of *Angelus Novus*, Paul Klee's "angel of history," smashed by wreckages of the past and pushed into "progress." If *I am time*, maybe somewhere between Krishna's "manifold forms of the universe united as one" and the James Webb Space Telescope looking "back" to "let there be light," can we be in the being, settle into a present progressive without the tense? *If you fall, I will catch you, I'll be waiting/ Time after time.*[24]

Maybe workshops and lunch with mayfield brooks or a couch conversation and french fries with Sage Ni'Ja Whitson or carefully constructed questions to Jennifer Monson were fertile humus in which I decomposed residual trainings and began the slow growth into the meaningful spaces of detritus, reclaimed single-use plastics, and chaotic installations in my ongoing *Tides Project*. Maybe Judy Hussie-Taylor sending me j. bouey's Instagram rumination on leaving Italy and our resulting chat and an online book club with (among others) devynn emory, Marýa Wethers, and Alicia ayo Ohs are the most meaningful threads in my work. But my work is not just my work for the stage, or the page, or the wage. I'll wager we find entanglement to be the emergent theory of organizing. We intersect in too many places, across all the times. So many of you are the stock in my stew. How could I not want sooner or later to remember you?

23 Oliver Burkeman, *Four Thousand Weeks: Time Management for Mortals* (New York: Farrar, Straus and Giroux, 2021); Elisabeth Tova Bailey, *The Sound of a Wild Snail Eating* (Chapel Hill, NC: Algonquin Books, 2016).

24 Cyndi Lauper, "Time after Time," 1983.

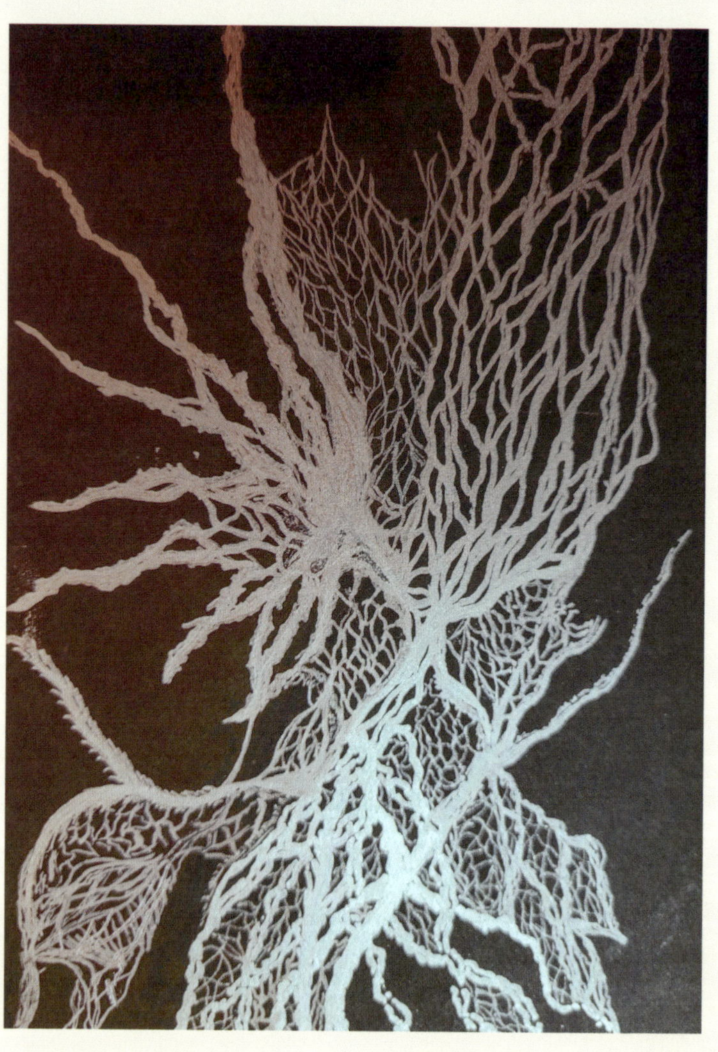

I just walked into the office of Paul Dennis, the chair of the Hunter College dance department, and said, *I have a fragile seedling of an idea that will need to be carefully tended.* Can a public MFA in dance in New York City serve as a pathway back to an integrated humanity for a planet in crisis? Can we Mother Tree this? Can we braid the sweetgrass[25] and invite Indigenous wisdom to soften the hard edges of scientific knowledge? Can we honor our entire ecosystem like the Haudenosaunee Thanksgiving Address?[26] Can we, at least, try to use dance to serve human wellness instead of serving supremacies? Can our bodies rest and move through space without fear of shame or assault, regardless of your aversion or desire? Can we return to our bodies, our breath, and become human, become animal, become tree kin, become ocean kin, become networked in a larger web of existence? Can we find ourselves sharing a history in a village of witnesses and weavers? Can someone ring the bell? It's time for nourishment.

25 Kimmerer, *Braiding Sweetgrass*.

26 Available at https://americanindian.si.edu/environment/pdf/01_02_Thanksgiving_Address.pdf.

Softly against jagged edges
The surface of a body as paint and concrete,
the surface of a painting as
skin and breath
Rest the cheek against the wall, feel
sharp points against membranes
Press upon it
Imprint a sylph
Merge
. merge .
. merge .
peel apart boundaries between we,
between me
scrape at reality
becoming and becoming, see?
coated in crumbled other
stripping the periphery
till molecules mingle
dusted and cover

you were there, i am there
you are there, i was there

somewhen
else

The Great Disappointment

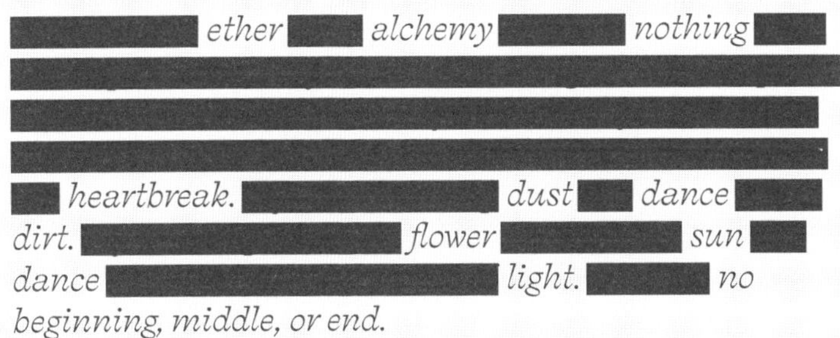

Long, long ago, life on Earth moved effortlessly for all living beings. Plants, animals, and humans lived together in appreciation of one another. They were united in their quest for survival and pleasure. Plants were the primary teachers on Earth. They could regenerate themselves, and they could sustain other species who ate their seeds, flowers, and stems. Some plants were fungal beings who could also feed on humans, animals, and insects. In death there was life. Plant teachers gleaned their pleasure from this delicious cycle of decomposition. Animals, humans, and insects revered the plants and their wisdom.

rooting and sky touching

Plants shared their knowledge of the land and the sky so that all sentient beings could understand how to reach up toward the light and root down into the ground. Reaching up toward the light brought growth. Rooting down brought nutrients from below. All beings on Earth were aware of this abundance and began to reach toward the light and root into the ground to honor what was given. This became a timeless dance—a common language of rooting and sky touching.

Discovery of gravitational pull and reaching toward the light became the dance of expansion for all beings. They were emulating their plant teachers. The tender pea plant with its knobby roots and climbing tendrils was the master teacher who guided humans and four-leggeds with perfecting their movement language. And so it was that human and nonhuman animals began each waking day with the dance of rooting and sky touching.

Bodily communication became so vast and euphoric that sometimes the humans would dance themselves to death. They always had large appetites for pleasure, which pleased their plant teachers. The four-leggeds were not so pleased. They saw something in humans that they could not recognize in themselves, and it frightened them. The plant teachers noticed the four-leggeds' displeasure and encouraged them to call a meeting with the humans.

competition, an aberration

One day, a conflict arose between the humans and the four-leggeds. After an extraordinary day of spontaneous rooting and sky touching, the humans dared the four-leggeds to outdance them! The dust rose under their voracious feet. They grabbed the air above like children chasing fireflies. They rolled around in the dirt. "Hey, four-leggeds, watch us dance!" they shouted. "We dare you to dance with the same speed and precision that we do!" The four-leggeds declined and rejected the humans' dare.

After the dare, relations began to sour between the humans and the four-leggeds. The four-leggeds felt disrespected by the humans' attitude of superiority. In reaction to the four-leggeds' dismissal of their dare, the humans called a meeting. In the meeting, they proposed that one human challenge one four-legged to a dance duel. The humans were intent on creating a new way of relating that they called competition. They wanted to be recognized for their prowess, *and* they wanted to test their new way of relating with the others. The humans' behavior confused the others because they felt that prowess was a given. This new way of relating that humans called competition broke group trust, and all they had ever had was trust. Their plant teachers taught them this.

Taken aback by the humans' proposal, the four-leggeds decided to retreat to the forest in protest, and some went to the sea. They couldn't imagine a world where they didn't work together, so they rejected the human proposal altogether. The humans asked the plant teachers to make the four-leggeds come back, but the plant teachers decided not to interfere. The humans became more and more aggressive with each passing day. They found pleasure in the challenge of competing, but over time this way of relating bred dissension and discord. They competed with one another relentlessly, threw their bodies against one another in brazen displays of strength, and raised their balled-up fists to the sky to show off their mastery. They slowly ceased participating in the rooting and sky-touching dances, and they stopped seeking counsel from the plant teachers. Instead, they relied only on themselves. They trained their bodies to move swiftly, quickly, and dangerously.

casting a spell

frozen time

The plant teachers grew weary of human aggression. In response, they cast a spell over the land. Growth ceased, and all went dormant. They called upon the heavens to usher in an excruciating chill that froze the Earth. Before long, the entire planet was blanketed in snow and ice.

The four-leggeds and sea creatures had been in regular communication with the plant teachers, so they knew how to prepare for the planetary freeze. They busied themselves with a variety of rooting and sky-touching dances that brought them an abundance of food. They discovered a new way of sleeping called hibernation. Meanwhile, the humans were too busy competing to consult with the plant teachers and therefore did not know how to hibernate when the freeze came. The humans relied on their own minds for information and forgot the dances of rooting and sky touching. Their fingers, which used to reach up for the light, turned into fists, and their feet, which used to root into the ground, were now kicking up dust and anger. This disappointed their plant teachers once again.

The human mind had been complex and brilliant, but once they lost their connection to the plant teachers, four-leggeds, insects, and other beings on Earth, they became unhinged, hierarchical, and aggressive. Humans lost their appetite for pleasure. They began to start wars among themselves. Survival became a game of predator and prey. This ushered in the Great Disappointment.

With the advent of the Great Disappointment, humans forgot what the plant teachers taught them. Humans forgot the interconnected dances of rooting and sky touching. Humans lost their memory of time before time. Humans lost hope. The human condition was plagued by an epidemic of heartbroken souls wandering the earth.

A Communion of Elders

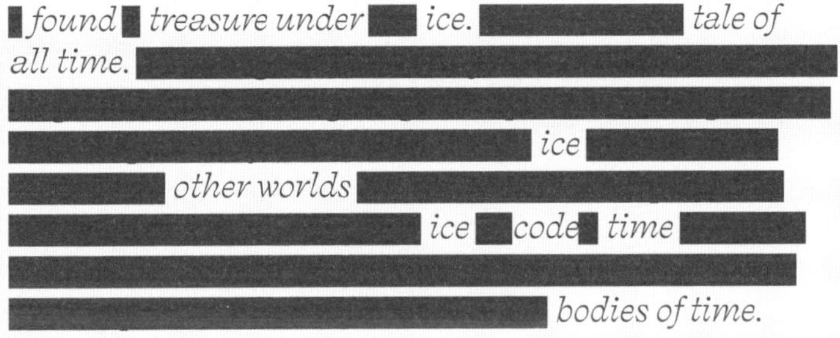
found treasure under ice. tale of all time.
ice
other worlds
ice code time
bodies of time.

We broke through the firmament effortlessly and swung into Earth's atmosphere with an assurance from those above that we would also be able to reach the depths of Earth's oceans with ease. As above, so below—or so we thought. It was not communicated to us that this venture to Planet Earth could not occur without permission from a council that called itself the Atlantic Elders. They were a motley crew of Neanderthals, radical ocean-dwelling expatriates, a community of seaweed, an assortment of marine mammals, and a collective of four-leggeds who wanted to be in on the conversation about why we had come to Earth. They greeted us with aplomb as we landed on what Earthlings call Antarctica.

Our elders, who reside within a different dimensional world—the seventh dimension—sent us to Earth at the request of the Atlantic Elders. Miraculously, through an alchemical process, the Atlantic Elders were able to pierce through the third dimension to the seventh dimension. We do not know how they accomplished this unforeseen feat, and they did not reveal their tactics. Before the Great Disappointment caused a global surge of heartbreak on Earth, the Atlantic Elders sent a message to our world.

It took centuries for our elders to receive the message from the Atlantic Elders because time is not compartmentalized in our world. Our elders were intrigued by the poetic nature of the request, which read something like this: "Please help us rearrange time and space so that a broader range of interspecies communication can occur on Earth. WE NEED HELP mending the epidemic of millions of broken hearts, resulting in large swaths of humans losing access to their imaginations and ability to create culture." The last line read, "Humans have forgotten how to dance."

The Atlantic Elders realized that without dance, humans had no real reason to exist outside of chaos, violence, and sadness. If bodies couldn't imagine movement and had no access to creativity, there was no motivation toward progress. Upon our arrival in Antarctica, the Atlantic Elders explained to us that, from the beginning of time, all beings on Earth survived through growth that involved movement—whether a seed sprouting, a bear hunting for salmon, or humans tilling the fields to grow food for their communities—and all movement was dance to all beings. The Atlantic Elders wanted to create a world where interspecies communication could occur, so that humans could learn back their imaginations and regain their memory of dance from species they thought were lesser than them. These so-called lesser species were the animals, insects, birds, and plants that had survived the Great Disappointment with their hearts and dances intact. Aided by earth, wind, fire, and water, the so-called lesser species had an incredible range of movement. They were far more adept at navigating a variety of land- and waterscapes—whether mountains, jungles, glaciers, or oceans.

The Atlantic Elders were convinced that movement and dance should never be compartmentalized or differentiated. They needed us to help calibrate Earth's rhythms with those of the human heart, so that humans could be tricked into dancing again by the beating of their own hearts. Since we were not visible to the human eye and had the capacity to shape-shift, we could assist in a rhythmic global recalibration of time and space. The Atlantic Elders told us that even though they had evolved during the time before history, they could not, on their own, align Earth's rhythms with those of the human heart. However, they could time travel, they were invisible to humans, and they remembered when movement and sound were primary modes of communication. They also remembered when there was no hierarchy among humans, animals, and plants. But they could not shape-shift as we could.

Humans were shrewd and valued their intelligence above all other beings on Earth. They constructed a narrative for themselves: their brains were equipped with the ability to exist beyond survival, to create great civilizations, and to progress into the future through industry and technology. This narrative nearly destroyed Earth and created a version of humanity that could not function without technology. Humans could no longer move on their own; they let other implements move them. What humans called progress, the Atlantic Elders called destruction. Humans were always delusional. Time and again, they let their intelligence override their intuition. The Atlantic Elders felt that dance was the most intrinsic amalgamation of intellect and intuition. Our task was to help humans create a physical and psychological bridge between intelligence and intuition.

Despite their overblown egos, humans were good collectors of information, and they kept written records of almost every sentient being on the planet in the Archive. The Atlantic Elders had no use for the Archive, but they did appreciate how thorough it was. We asked what caused them to reject the Archive, and they told us that humans had put too much faith in words. They wanted humans to reclaim their sensory abilities and perhaps tap into different ways of seeing what the Atlantic Elders called clairvoyance. According to them, the Archive had ushered in the Great Disappointment, which led to the heartbreak epidemic. The Archive also chronicled the Great Disappointment.

In addition to calibrating the rhythms of the human heart to that of the Earth, the Atlantic Elders needed us to assist them in helping humans open up their hearts again (so many broken hearts—so, so many). The only way to do this was through dance, touch, sensing, and being with plants, animals, and other beings. Humans also needed help reaching across time to ancestors who lived before the creation of history. The Atlantic Elders felt that interspecies relationality and communion with prehistoric ancestors could be achieved only by breaking through the time-space continuum. This would give humans a portal into a time when everything danced, a time before language, a time before the Archive. For the Atlantic Elders, this process required a period of osmosis that would allow the human brain to unthink itself and merge with other sentient beings and elemental forces, reminding it of what it felt like to exist without compartmentalized time and thought. Humanity needed to be completely immersed in a world of sensation.

Since we were beings without bodies, we understood the immensity of our task. Our elders suggested that we shape-shift into human form to better understand the human body. The most important thing, they said, is that you learn how they move. In our dimension, there is no compartmentalization of movement and stillness. Everything is everything. We function as bodies without substance or form.

To shape-shift into humans, we had to visualize every aspect of human form, evolution, and development. This became the most strenuous endeavor. We were fortunate to discover that the human heart's rhythm could guide us in our development as humans—from embryo to infant, from infant to child, and from child to adult.

The Archive

a dancer. history. I
move water, earth
My body is not
Dance history
Create
fables. stories.

Antarctica proved a great place for us to land. The Archive had been buried under the snow for probably more than a millennium. The Atlantic Elders guided us to it. Some of the Neanderthal Atlantic Elders were familiar with the landscape of Antarctica from their days living in the Ice Age. They located the Archive by consulting the ice and listening to how it echoed as it cracked. Antarctica quieted us, and we were ready when the ice spoke and told us the story of the Great Disappointment.

As beings without bodies, we found the Archive a useful tool for understanding why the Great Disappointment had caused so many broken hearts. During the time of timelessness, when humans, animals, insects, and plants all used dance as their primary method of communication, their hearts were intact. We wanted to shape-shift into humans with strong hearts, so we imagined what it would feel like to have a human body in the time of timelessness. Before our shape-shifting transformation, we imagined how our human bodies would feel in the act of reaching up toward the light and rooting into the ground. We studied the growth processes of plants in all stages of development, from seed to fruit, and it became clear to us that the origin of all life on the planet was something extremely simple—microbes. Then the Atlantic Elders confirmed this, letting us know that all living things on Earth most likely originated from some kind of bacteria not visible to the human eye.

We realized that reintroducing humans to their prehistoric dances would bring them back into a space of ancestral memory. If they tapped into this past, they could resurrect their latent power of clairvoyance, transporting themselves back to a time before the heartbreak. Then we shape-shifters could help them imagine a future filled with bodies that danced again.

Timelessness

Prehistory. Time before time. *(We danced.)* Shape-shift now, then, and later. Remember what has been broken. Forget what has been broken. Revisit ice, stone, water, and metal. What came before thought? What came before language? *(We danced.)* What came before necessity? What came before cultivation? What came before incessant digging? What came before control? *(We danced.)* What came before freedom and ideas? What came before now? What comes later?

Body roots into the ground. Body sleeps. Body yields to the earth. *(I dance.)* Body lies flat. Body turns on its side. Body breathes. *(I dance.)* Body reaches toward the light. Body rises. Body balances. Body erupts. Body bounces. Body explodes into a million shards of glass. Body hurts. *(I dance.)* Body recovers. Body heals. Body dies. Body decomposes. *(I dance.)*

12

REMEMORY of a spine arching upward toward the sky.

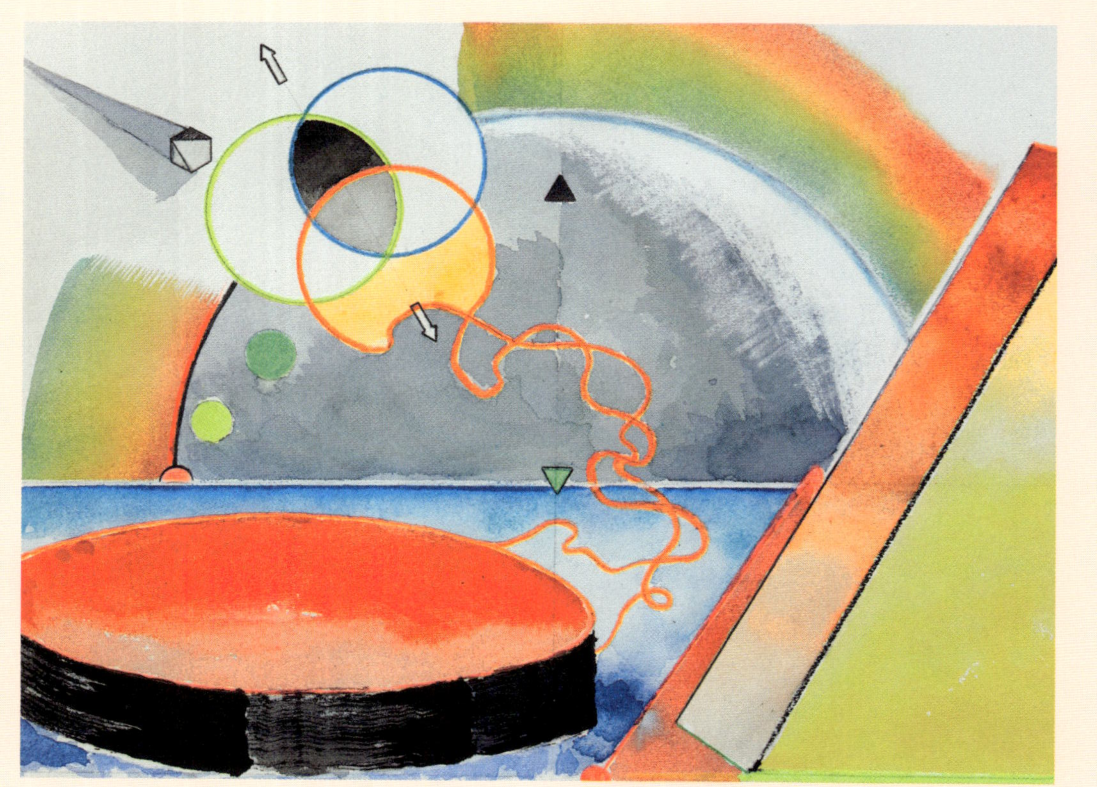

One long spine. *(They dance.)*

Light finds SPINE centuries old.

Whale spine carries Archive. *(We dance.)*

Skeletons and bones tell the STORY.

An Archive of MARROW. *(I dance.)*

An Archive of BONES.

Epilogue: Present Time

RIP Rockaway "Baby" Sperm Whale

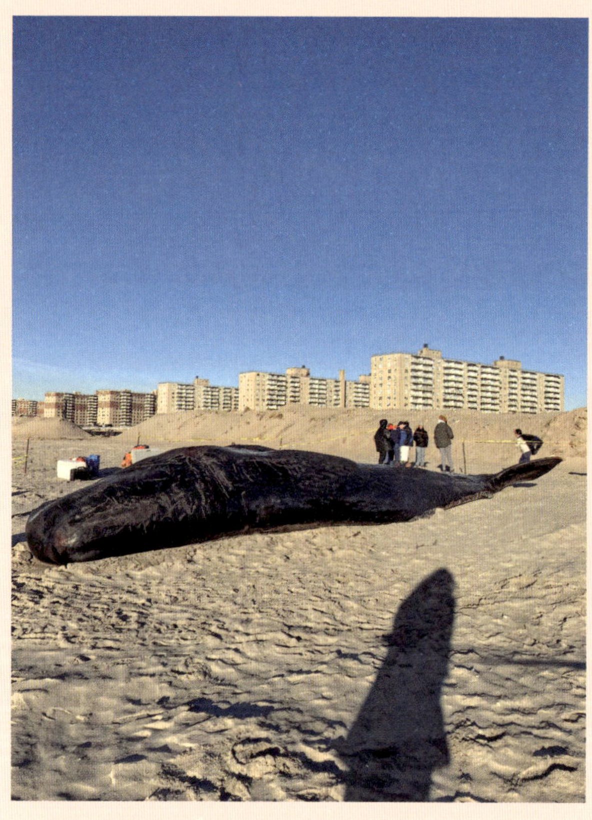

This 👆 is the Rockaway Beach whale who passed away on December 12, 2022, after several attempts to save it. The shadow is mine.

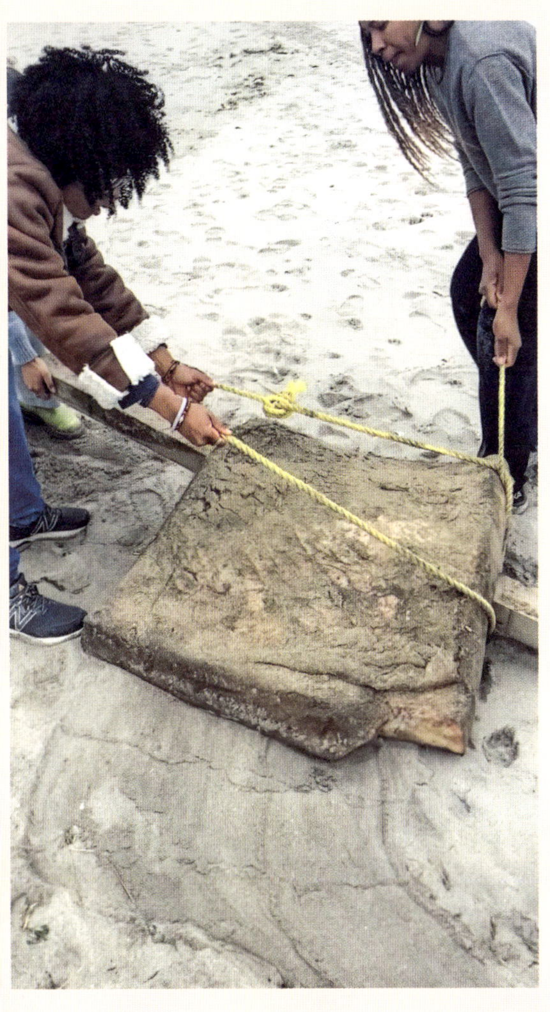

After it died, the "experts" performed a necropsy on the whale. They buried it, and pieces of its body resurfaced on Rockaway Beach. When we found it, the whale flesh was stuck behind a human-made sand dune from a construction site, and we decided to return it to the sea. It was so heavy that four of us couldn't pick it up, so we rigged it to a wooden plank and some rope and dragged it back to the shore.

As the ocean received the whale's remains, I laid my body down on its flesh and for a brief moment danced a small dance and said goodbye.

If dance is simultaneously a transmission, a collaboration, a collision, a collusion, an encounter where a ripple from behind the belly button threads its way to the edge of a body's border, where the hairs on the skin stand on edge in the space between another body's edge, charged and reaching out toward the other, I want to consider a history of this charge. I want to consider collaborations, collisions, collusions, transmissions.

My history of dance must begin with my first collaboration, the dance with my mother, a duet attuned to our mutual heartbeats, a dance in the womb, a song in the key of water.

Multicellular eukaryotic period:

My mother becomes two, so her body is the site of an embryonic entanglement, our first movement phrase. The cell holds genetic material like offerings in an archive. It is a book listing an endless trail of begets. It is being written as it is read. This cell is dividing and splitting, absorbing and shedding with every mitochondrial aspiration. The binding of the book is thickening and cracking wide open with the weight of each new page, each new possibility—a grandfather's eye color, your grandmother's loud arguments with the multiple voices that only she can hear, your possible future child's fixation on sucking the salt off a sunflower husk before discarding the seed. All of this shifting, repetition, and change is a vibration that is also recalling and forgetting, that is a future constantly emerging, entangled in and stretching away from the past.

When you are suspended between the
memory of all that came before and
dreams that are sparks for a multitude of
possible futures, this is the first lesson
in understanding how a dance is made.

Isn't this first dance a collaboration?
This dance with my mother, a duet
attuned to our mutual heartbeats,
a song in the key of water?

Cellular memory is simultaneously a residue of past bodies and a prelude to future bodies. I imagine an acidic and salty silt that churns and gives rise to an emergent dance that quotes previous choreographies and invents new movements.

One score emerging from the silt comes from the girl who will become my mother in a village in the South East region of Nigeria, who runs the fastest and whose dance seems the most mischievous because it takes unpredictable turns. It is the *egedege* she's mastered. Her torso is slightly forward, her hips are activated in a clear antecedent to twerking, her feet are ancestors to samba. When she drops suddenly, gravity does not win. Her face is placid, while her torso and legs are having a circular and raucous conversation with the drums.

The girl watches the boy who can captivate you with his dance—particularly when he does the dance that mimics the way a large and beautiful bird moves, swooping in for prey, fluttering its wings. He won't do this dance without the drum telling him exactly what to do. (This boy will become my father. And I've asked him to show me the dance, but he says he can't without the drum's instruction.) This dance is called the *ubo ogazi*, translated roughly, by him, as "the instrument that the eagle dances to." (He can't remember the exact name of the bird in English, so he calls it an eagle. It is actually a guinea fowl.) He will leave the village a young man and take his dance across the ocean, replacing the guinea fowl with an eagle. And why not, when he will dance in the land that has chosen the soaring eagle as its symbol? There will be drums, and he will dance to raise money for his people's suffering during a civil war.

When the young woman crosses the ocean, she brings the *egwu obi*, the dance of her mother and her mother's sisters. It means "the dance of the heart." This is a slower dance than the *egedege*. She drops low into a deep bend and slowly winds her way back up toward the sky. Her arms are suspended laterally from her sides, softly turning, a soft twist from her shoulders to her wrists. She is all curves and wind. And even

when she is not low to the ground,
her knees are bent, the small of her back
is arched, and her hips draw parabolas
behind her. She dances alone and on the
steps of the United Nations; she makes
her heart dance, raising money
for the Biafran Relief Organization.

Not being there on the ground, in her
country, during the worst of the war and
the resulting famine, seeing the pain
from a distance, she does not feel grief
at a distance—this is dance work done
to keep her heart from breaking—

and
breaking.

Dancing to songs in the key of concrete,
a minor key:

Swaggering onto the playground with
cardboard and boom box, the boys—
they are mostly boys—lay the cardboard
down on the concrete, set down the
boom box, raise the volume to the max,
and go into a rhythmic skip, moving
side to side in a quick cross step, like

warming up an engine and getting ready to drive. And even with all this dance of getting ready, it's still a shock as they propel themselves into a coiled inversion. The palms of their hands hit the ground first. Even though it looks like their heads will crack against the concrete, which no cardboard can protect against, they hover before touching the ground, bending and twisting and turning, like bobbling extensions of their neck—a rejoinder to gravity, an argument against bone as anything harder than the soft, pliable skeleton in utero.

Double Dutch seems saner to me.

Another collaboration that requires at least three people—two to turn, one to jump. And then a rope. Turning two ropes at a time, rhythm. When I learned to turn, I felt I understood everything I needed to know about double Dutch. Two ropes in two hands, working in a kind of canon with each other. The turn comes from the wrists and the hands, not the arms. There was a music you should hear to keep the ropes from "kissing"—the name we have for the tangling of rope, usually when the rope turner falls out of the canon's rhythm. We always blame the turners when the ropes kiss. The accusation flies from the jumper's mouth: "You turn doublehanded!" This means that, even for a moment, your two hands have betrayed you and fallen into the mal-rhythm, where you're turning the two separate ropes at the same time, not in the steady iambic rhythm required. You had a speech deficit where your two tongues got entangled and tied up in each other, making jumping between them impossible. That's why we prefer an extra-long telephone cord that we can fold into two ropes, because insulated wire holds its arc, even with a turner who might accidentally fall into a moment of doublehandedness when the ropes are going at high speed. As a turner, you pulse, moving side to side, in time with the rhythm of the ropes' canon, and you watch the jumper with eyes wide and ablaze, attuned to any subtle body shifts that the jumper might make to signal the need to slow down or speed up. These prime three, alert to one another, dancing with one another, the ropes making an orbit around the jumper—the hope is to sustain this rigorous bliss for as long as possible.

And I don't call it bliss, but what else could it be? What word could describe the feeling of being with one another, not knowing what's coming next, of only attending to what the moment needs in our triad, with our adrenaline pumping, our heartbeats racing, all of us fluid and pulsing together in a music of our own making? I loved the "pop-ups," when, instead of alternating laterally from left foot to right, the jumps were straight up and vertical, the standard form when turning with one rope. But to pop-up in double Dutch is to time your leap so that you don't hit the rope arcing above your head while not stepping on the rope hitting the ground beneath you. It is suspended and in flight at the same time. You would think the unyielding concrete we play on were a sprung floor.

But the spring is in us. Springing like coiled wire. I make sure my rope is always in my book bag during the school year or twined around my arm in the summertime, ready to play wherever and whenever two other people are ready to sweat. We are always, at the very least, a trio that could evolve into a quartet or a septet. On a long, hot summer night, the number of us in our gathering and growing pulse is a thrill. We are a world.

Gathering.

Dancing to songs in the key of being.
All of us. Together.

It is the mid-1980s, and we must have gone to every Nigerian (Igbo) wedding in the tristate area for the past decade. I've attended at least one in each of my twelve years, haven't I? The reception is my favorite part. There is always a moment when a women's group dances in a procession into the wedding hall, subtle footwork, knees slightly bent, hips unbothered and unhurried, loose. The women want you to watch them, but they seem to be more interested in their own pleasure, as if to say, "Yes, we're celebrating the spiritual union of two families, but we are also celebrating how good it can feel to inhabit our own bodies, these bodies that may bear the fruit of this union, watch this miracle that is our body." It is grounded murmuration.

I don't know who leads or follows or which direction they are going in, but I am mesmerized.

As they dance, the other adults in the room start to "spray" the dancers with money—one dollar, twenty dollars. Or maybe some especially affluent person has a stack of fifty-dollar bills in hand, shuffling money at the dancers as if shuffling cards into the air, a croupier with no table and no sense, just making it rain. The children are tasked with picking up the money because the dancers cannot be bothered to interrupt their flow for something as mundane as picking up cash. And any child who thought they could pocket an extra ten-dollar bill or just one dollar always seems to be caught and quickly brought to heel. But a child can also dance, and if that child starts to evince signs of exertion, or if a sheen of sweat surfaces on the child's forehead, maybe they will be sprayed with money.

Dancing vigorously for a long time without any overt appearance of effort, only a trace of it in the subtle, dewy shine of your face, always elicits praise.

And attention.

Attunement.

Dancing in the key of roiling quiet.

I see Min Tanaka at Performance Space 122, and I can't find a single word for what I am witnessing or what is happening in my body. I find a flood of words that then recedes. He is a young boy who became an ancient crone. He has no eyes and then he does have eyes, but they are somewhere in his throat and he can see only through his gaping mouth. And then he is a mirror. I am watching him and, at the same time, falling into some unfathomable universe within myself.

I go to Min Tanaka's Body Weather farm in Hakushu, Japan, joining dancers, historians, artists, writers, and "company men." (The latter are mostly Japanese, in their thirties or forties, from the corporate world, and the most mysterious to me—they bring an edge of suffering to the work they do, though it may just be that in the high heat of the noonday summer sun, moving through the aerobic floor work at the beginning of every workshop, they are in fact suffering.)

We all have come together to investigate the "weather" within our bodies with a liberating rigor.

I am the only Black woman, and my desire to attune to the Body Weather dance practice and the community of people gathered for that purpose is coupled with a quiet and growing sense of alienation throughout my time there.

The work requires a rigorous and sustained exploration through an inner life rich with images that can arouse a depth of sensation and serve as a springboard to move. I have to be able to shut my outside eye. Paradoxically, as a Black woman, my survival depends on keeping that eye open and alert. I knew I would begin this practice—touching the edge of being in myself and attuning to the world outside of me from the world within me—but that work will not end here. It might never end.

I lie down in shallow streams to
understand how to partner with water.
I climb a tree for the first time as my
exercise partner stands at its base calling
images up to me: "garden growing
from the crown of your head," "snake in
your spine," "intestines spilling out of your
splayed open stomach," "child feet."
And I make more: "ants marching up and
down the outer edges of my arms,"
"spider trying to crawl into my right ear,"
"back rib cage opening wide as a crow
tries to break free from my lungs"—
all of this to awaken a sensing body. How
deeply can one dance from the inside?

What sense do I make about that part of my day spent finding my way along rows of cabbage, squatting and looking for worms eating through the leaves? When I find worms, I pluck them off and squish them between my fingers. I wipe their remains in the earth. I am a murderer of worms and a protector of cabbage. Through stalking worms, I develop my capacity to squat for hours at a time. I feel clean. My skin is baking but protected under a layer of dust. I ride a bike everywhere. As I walk across a rice paddy, I see a snake slither past me at lightning speed. I feel the acute charge of the possibility of an encounter.

Welcoming encounters to dance not just with people but with the earth: the soles of feet pressing into damp soil, toes burrowing into the ground like tree roots.

Min leads us to a stream after an hour of floor work. We lie down, sweat soaking through our clothes to mingle with the stream's fresh water. He tells us not to turn nature into some distant object we take pictures of, judge as to its beauty, and never touch. He makes it clear that we are idiots if we don't understand nature to be as alive as we are. I think he wants us to allow ourselves to be moved by nature; he is inviting us to give ourselves over to a literal dance with this shallow stream, allowing wind and water to take the lead.

I am learning to find the impulse to dance at the point where the interior imagination and the external living world collide. When this dance started, how it will progress, and when it might end are not the questions to engage just then.

But the question of losing oneself in a performance practice or being at the edge of getting lost in a dance remains. If you get lost, where do you go? And how do you come back? Who will find you? What do you return to? Is a performance or dance practice about mastery and control in every moment? Is it about mastering yourself? Or is it about mastering the ability to wander into a somatic and psychic landscape that is wild and overgrown and in constant flux?

I am looking to wander through
the overgrowth.
I am looking to be in the inner wild
and still sense its edges.

Dancing to songs in a multitude of keys and questions. Dance as a map through a multitude of questions that dance in you.
Ralph Lemon, the mapmaker.
Come home Charley Patton (2004) is dance in the space of memory, dance as shaky historical mapping, dance as grief, as a history of place and relation.

Ralph gives us these keywords to make a dance phrase: "Wind... Ground (Hallow)... Memorial (Counter)... Water, Horse (Animal)... Fury... Flurry... Praise... Rapture... Spiral... Circle... Spiral... Surrender... Courage... Trust... Shaky Elegance."[1]

1 Ralph Lemon, *Come home Charley Patton* (Middleton, CT: Wesleyan University Press, 2013), 186–87.

Is Ralph quietly searching for a way back to the salt churn of an embryonic Black body entangled in and shaped by the violence of capture and resistance in the United States of America? If Ralph is trying to dance in the space where his postmodern dance/art practice (a particular formal body liberation) collides with the density and complication of race (an ongoing struggle for bodily autonomy), how do you dance alongside him in it?

I did not know of Trisha Brown. I did not know that she made *Planes* and *Falling Duet I* in 1968, the same year the Civil Rights Act was passed. It included the Fair Housing Act. I did not know that as Brown was constructing dance that broke free from the spatial constraints and entrenched vocabularies of concert dance—challenging even the constraints of gravity—Black folks were fighting to break free of the limitations of laws that were written to keep them impoverished and keep their bodies "in place."

Come home Charley Patton is the first and last time I am asked if I am open to dancing under the full force of an open fire hose. I said that I was not okay with that. We watch the documentary series *Eyes on the Prize* (1987), and we all see a young man fall and get back up and seem to dance his resistance to the violence of white supremacy, and we are amazed.[2] In the performance, Ralph does this dance. Another collaborator, Darrell Jones, enters the space downstage of the hosing, falling and flying up in relation to Ralph falling and getting back up. To me, this phrase is an active choreography of transmission happening in real time, from the young man in *Eyes on the Prize* through to Ralph and then on to Darrell.

2 *Eyes on the Prize*, episode 4, "No Easy Walk: 1961–1963," directed by Callie Crossley and James A. DeVinney, first broadcast on PBS on February 11, 1987.

This work ends with a phrase we called "Ecstasy." In it, Djédjé Djédjé Gervais, Darrell Jones, Gesel Mason, David Thomson, and I worked with Ralph to map out a wild course of collisions that seemed to be the memory of all the dance phrases in the performance. We were dancing within and beyond the memory of Wind, Ground (Hallow), Memorial (Counter), Water, Horse (Animal), Fury, Flurry, Praise, Rapture, Spiral, Circle, Spiral, Surrender, Courage, Trust, all with a certain Shaky Elegance.

Our gestural phrases make me think of an early sprout breaking through the seed and taking root. I felt myself take root, unravel, and blossom along a new trajectory in a cycle seeding a multitude of futures.

(the Efflorescence of) Walter.[3]

3 Ralph Lemon, *(the Efflorescence of) Walter*, May 11–June 23, 2007, the Kitchen, New York.

Walter Carter's centenarian stillness is poised suspension. His dance is with the past, present, and future. He is the haunted interstellar traveler in Bentonia, Mississippi. He knows why the Delta clay has a blood tint. But he knows the darkness that seems to swallow up the road should also be read as a celestial premonition. His feet are planted firmly on the ground and his hands clasped behind his back. The most pressing question is, "When will he take flight"?

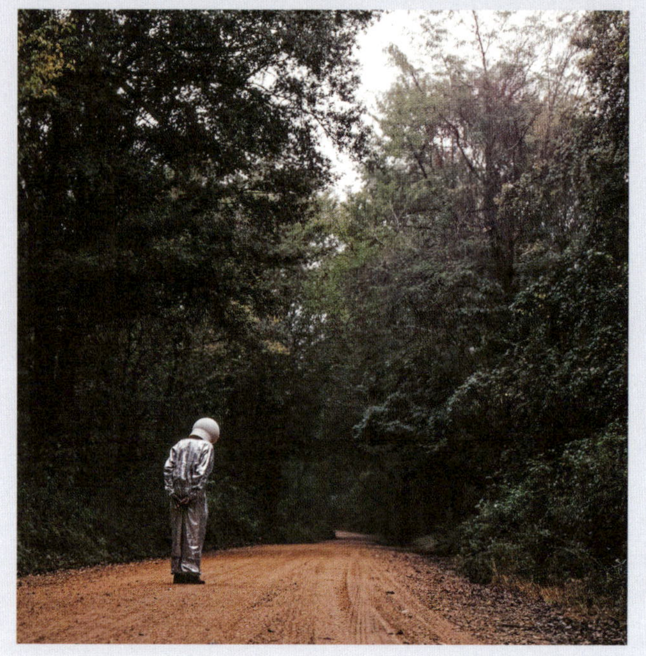

I long for the two-spirit dances (and language
and ways) of my Indigenous ancestors.
Weren't your people colonized at some point, too?
What were their first dances?

Here is a gesture.

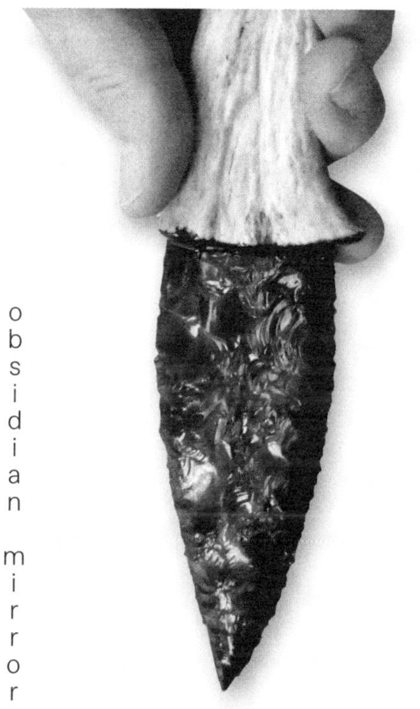

To remind us of the truths/violences everywhere
and in all times. A ward against (uncritical) nostalgia,
against the "utopic" that hides the dystopic.

Javier

2

How We Arrive

The dance began tomorrow.
The children are already dreaming the rhythms,
its heart, incubating.

Some for the pavement
moment before class
Some for the
night-club floor
fully
fleshed,
their
sinews
compressed
encoded
in the
star carbon
Seeds we
sow today
plaza soil
Some for the mission

Some for the pavement
moment before class
Some for the
night club floor
fully
fleshed,
their
sinews
compressed
encoded
in the
star carbon
Seeds we
sow today
plaza soil
Some for the mission

We are our ancestors. Literally. The matter of our flesh is
reconstituted from our many nonhuman relations…
the more-than-human… the ancient ones… our ancestors
in us… This is what so many of our origin stories tell us.
From this flows much of our original instructions…

Seeds carried on the winds…
Seeds carried (farthest, across time) by storms…
Lightning, bringing fire before rain
Seeds sprouted (only) by flame

Blessed be we who remember their songs
from the future.
Blessed be we who

imagine

ancestors' voices come from tomorrow, the past that
pulls us forward…

So You and I May Begin Well (Again)

The imposter (syndrome) says "hola."

God, I hope I can keep it short this time.

I write this from Yelamu (San Francisco, stolen Ramaytush Ohlone lands), where I have lived, played, and worked for about four years, with eleven more living in different parts of the Bay Area. Ohlone peoples of many bands have called this land home for thousands of years, and many continue fighting for cultural recognition, rematriation of their lands, and restoration of cultural land stewardship.

I am the mixed-race, detribalized descendant of Piru and Tigua Pueblo Native nations.

Most of my blood is mixed European,
and my Frésquez name traces to Jan Frisch.
(Spelling?... does it matter? ^This settler's^
legacy lives on in my name.)
Jan was a Flemish man who settled in
New Mexico during Spanish colonial rule
in the 1600s and changed his name to
Juan Fresco. Across the centuries, "Fresco"
evolved into "Frésquez."

I grew up in El Paso, Texas.

I don't know the names for the area before
the conquistador Hernán Cortés showed up
and decided it was Spain's. I don't know any
"fully Native" ancestors' names...

My father's family's land, a ten-acre cotton farm in Socorro, Texas, has been in the Frésquez family for generations. It is where I grew up with my father and, for some years, with my grandmother Cecilia Candelaria Frésquez. The Frésquez family is mixed

and descended from Piru Pueblo Natives.
The Candelarias are mixed descendants of
Tigua Pueblo Natives.

Everyone in my family that I knew as
I was growing up was some kind of
devout Catholic. Not much Native cultural
grounding to speak of there.
Also, I didn't work the land much, except for the
little vegetable garden my father had us start
once or twice. We didn't grow traditional crops
or tend the garden in a traditional way.
Even so, I learned to put my hands in the
soil. When I swam in the drainage ditch,
the water with all its agrochemicals caressed
my body as it slowly seeped into the Hueco
Bolson, the enormous aquifer beneath us.
At times, I walked along the land and
breathed the air contemplatively, making
dances in my head and quietly within my
skin. It all formed me, and I learned much
from it. Wouldn't it be disrespectful of me
to deny that? I try to honor it.

The Tigua's reservation, Ysleta del Sur Pueblo,
is widely known and federally recognized.
I grew up maybe two miles from that.
The Piru don't have federal recognition, and I always
thought they had little to no sense of community,
common identity, or traditional culture.

Then I looked up Piru on Wikipedia and
learned a lot more. LOL. For starters, the
tribe's name is spelled P-i-r-o by many,
including the anthropologists and whoever
made it Wikipedia official.

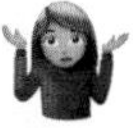

As a queer person of Indigenous descent doing decolonial cultural work in community with two-spirits, I identify as two-spirit. For several years, I supported the Bay Area American Indian Two-Spirit Powwow as a volunteer on the powwow committee; after that, one of the committee's cochairs at the time encouraged me to start "representing."

I will likely never have children. Still, I hope that my refusal to accept colonial amnesia and my work in Indigenous communities will leave a trail of seeds behind me.

Those seeds

.

may not be

.

for me

.

to sow

.

.

.

so?

I may never be affirmed or recognized as
"Native enough" by some. I may never
deeply learn my ancestral languages and
dances, be recognized as a part of a tribe,
or have a blood quantum that means
enough to my family members to bring
them into Indigenous practices and
community. Nonetheless, I refuse to let
my Native ancestors and cultures die (an
absolute genocide) with me.

Also FUCK THIS exercise in self-doubt and
performative self-revelation/authentication.
The ice caps are melting,
the wildfires are spreading,
climate-induced chaos is coming,
and every last mutt, mestizo, mixed, resilient-
descendant-resisting-erasure among us needs to
start healing our world!
Now!

We must all begin to remember, with honesty.

Tecpatl for (Y)our Remembering[1]

We live in a time of escalating storms. Of empires and social orders crumbling as social inequality and the natural world's human-made disequilibria foment "chaos."

By "chaos," we mean possibility.

A storm was my first dance teacher. Storms past, present, and future stir in me, in my imaginings.

For me, to write about the origins of two-spirit dance is to tap a storm of voices all deserving to be heard in a world designed to ignore, misinterpret, and silence them. To learn two-spirit history of any kind, I must wade through anthropology documenting slaughter . . . that echoes today . . . a spiral that oscillates out from our bodies through how we gender, exploit, and control them . . . and to the lands and how we "own," gender, mine, and "manage" them.

One problem with writing anything down is that (we imagine) it's supposed to be right/clear/true across time. But I'm an emergent being in an emergent community, with emerging and constantly contested senses of identity. Identities are not reclaimed without

so

much

work.

And perhaps nothing I say now will

remain "true" for long

1 "Tecpatl is not only a [obsidian] dagger that cuts, flays, and wounds but a scalpel that opens and heals, a tongue that speaks sharply and accurately, an artifact of knowledge, wisdom, and experience...not focused on attacking (I am already strong there) but on healing, opening, and creating new notes/artifacts/dances/expressions/texts for use later." P. Don'Té Cuauhtémoc (Two-spirit Mexica dancer, choreographer, and vogue scholar), "Monsoon," in "Map of Slight Askew," *Loculus Journal*, no. 1 (January 2020), 6, https://www.loculuscollective.com.

And when thinking in English, well, we're…thinking in English, the language of the Angles…Far too much of the world now imagines itself through English. And (we imagine) what we read expresses something true about the "author." I'm not interested in writing like that. I don't think or tell stories in a line.

I'm not interested in one (line of) conversation,
one imaginary.
This conversation deserves to be stormed.

So, storm that I am, I'm trying something else…
Will you try—

You may want to read this paragraph in a mirror.
Indigenous fine print\your pre-tecpatl trigger warning:
Continuing to read this work constitutes consent to exposure to unsettling thoughts, memories, imaginings, emotional triggering, dreams, nightmares\heightened pattern matching, imaginative flights of fancy, projecting, projections, and every manner of popping your bubble that tends to happen when we really "decolonize" our "selves." Aho!?

—with me?

I will not be civil(ized) or "coherent." I will not imagine in (straight) line(s). I write against the slaughter, and I am not alone.
Aho?

First Dancer

First being of the origin of dance,
they who can dance all the music at once.

And one (gaze) could only perceive parts of the dance
at a time depending where one (gaze) focused.

Gazing upon them,
one's perspective and scale of frame illuminated
the dance in its various layers,
correlating the parts of action, feeling
the energies of impetus,
the percussive interactions,
resonances and antagonisms (musically).
Here a melody,
there
the fifth harmony,
there the counter tempo rhythm.

When I am most alive, most attuned, dancing
to my fullest, I feel the music dancing me...
all the music...dancing all of me. When I
share this dance in front of others, it often
overwhelms, and I've been told I'm doing too
much, that it "doesn't fit" (with the cultural
or social space)...It "takes up too much
space"...even when dancing (my cultures)
small but fully I take up a lot of space. But I
don't apologize unless I do harm...

Then the first dancer was split into many things.
Kaleidoscopic. Crystalline.

cogito ergo sum(?)

Spectral in vivisection.

Oye! You!

Zoom in

and

zoom

out!

(a simple exercise to imagine the first dancer)

a simple exercise to notice harm and critically question how we define *harm*.

How many more firsts have there been?
How many billions of bodies encountering each other
and the pulse of time?

To abstract it is to imagine it, and if we must imagine
the beginning, then we must imagine a beginner...
so you see how we immediately have choices to make?...

Who are your peoples?
How did they dance first?
How did their first dances end?

Maybe it matters more to imagine why a first
dance ends. Sure, maybe the dancer's body got
tired, or maybe that person was stilled by shame,
or maybe they danced themself off a cliff

.

.

.

and took the dance
with them into
the afterlife.

But I painfully find it much easier to believe that
the first dance was silenced by someone who
hated the dance(r).

By "dance" I also mean "chaos"
and "possibility".

Let's zoom in…

Jacqueline Shea Murphy has documented a long history of settler-colonists in the United States and Canada banning Native American dances and killing or imprisoning Native dancers of all ages across the centuries. Frequently, missionaries and government officials charged with managing/subduing Native American communities decried sexual "perversion" in ceremonies involving dance, projecting their own Christian ideas of monogamy and the sex-and-gender binary onto complex, ancient, and sophisticated practices[2]

and sometimes, simply innocent moments of joy and celebration.

2 Jacqueline Shea Murphy, *The People Never Stopped Dancing* (Minneapolis: University of Minnesota Press, 2007), 93-94.

How often do you find yourself distrusting LGBTQ2S+ people in your community/family? Do you trust them with children? And with the same kinds of family responsibilities that "straight" family members have?

Many Native dances were systematically eradicated as a part of the United States and Canada's ongoing efforts to "'civilize'—and thereby save—a dying people by incorporating Native people (who would then no longer be Indian) into the state."[3] So it'll come as no surprise that war dances and other dances understood to stir up aggression were also targeted. Not until the American Indian Religious Freedom Act of 1978 were many of these Native dances permissible under US law.

3 Ibid., 30.

Yes, the same Religious Freedom Act that the current majority-conservative US Supreme Court uses to justify the denial of services to LGBTQ2S+ by religious people.

And, honey, the darker and poorer and more out you are, the more you know this part specifically allows white (and white-aspiring or adjacent) people to discriminate against Brown, Black, Yellow, and Red queers.

People not too long ago used to fear dances.
To the NIMBYs out there: not too far away from you, there is, today, a dance form that would terrify you when it happens, encircled by the folks who invented it…
Maybe you can already think of what dance…

Don't seek it out!

I mean, maybe you can think of *who* dances like that…

Don't seek them out!

Don't seek it out, don't seek them out, unless you first check your privilege, check your worldview, check your whole world at the curb.

Ha!  #reverseOntologicalViolence 🧿

See to *avoid romanticizing the first dancers*, don't we have to imagine the violence of (or at least around) the first dance?

That's what I have to do to ask the question of how dance began for my people…

I have to wade through an anthropology that documents slaughter…

I'm interested in the complete and diasporic histories of queer dances and what could potentially be "Queer Dance."

I want to know the first dance of my Indigenous ancestors, the dance that I would do (then and now), the one that would fit the complexity of gender and sexuality that flows in me. "Male" dances are too painful. Across the male socialization of my childhood and adolescence, they made my mind and spirit sick.

Painting her nails obsidian black, she says, "Besides,
to only imagine Indigenous dances as gendered
within a binary simply lacks… imagination."💅

I want to learn third-gender words, roles, lifeways, and cultural practices of the Piro and the Tigua.

(Respectfully—if there were/are any)
I don't (even) know the third genders or
names of queer identities of my tribe, or if
they existed before the great forgetting.
Tongva two-spirit elder L. Frank Manriquez
calls ^it "the great contamination."

So, I ask you, what if the first Indigequeer, two-spirit, LGBTQIA++ dance was horizontal? What if it involved writhing, austerely ecstatic bodies squirming over one another?

Yummmmm.

It's certainly an evocative image . . . in my mind, with all the joy and healing I've had in experiences like it today, it is a good imagining.

It's a relevant imagining to these pages,

for you,
because of how much it evokes the historical reality of the *end* of this dan

ce for so many two-spirit dancers,

two-spirit people.

Behold the violent end of a two-spirit horizontal dance…[4]

258 GLQ: A JOURNAL OF LESBIAN AND GAY STUDIES

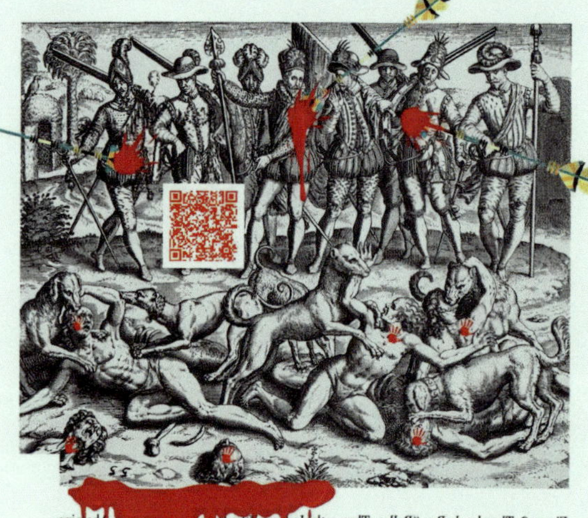

4 Arrows, blood, and QR code added by the author with ancient Canva Pro technology. #creativelicense.

Figure 2. Theodor de Bry, "Balboa Throws the Ind[illegible]ans Who H[illegible] Abomina[illegible] Crime of Sodomy to Be Torn to Bits by Dogs," eng[illegible]ving from [illegible]é de las Ca[illegible]as, *Narratio regionum Indicarum per Hispanos quosd[illegible]m deuestatarum [illegible]rissima* ([illegible]ankfurt: De Bry and Saurii, 1598)

one dog was worth fifty soldiers in subduing the Nat[illegible]es.[14] On September 23, 1513, the explorer Vasco Nuñez de Balboa came on about forty indigenous men, all dressed as women, engaged in what he called "preposterous Venus." He commanded his men to give the men as "a prey to his dogges," and the men were torn apart alive.[15] Coren states matter-of-factly that "these dogs were considered to be mere weapons and sometimes instruments of torture."[16] By the time the Spaniards

By holding this historical drawing up to a mirror, you can read who set the mastiffs on our queer ancestors and why. The image contains a seed I'll return to later.

If you are two-spirit or LGBTQ2SIA++, or an accomplice of indigequeers, and Indigenous creatures everywhere, the QR code links to a dance offering that is available to you whenever you need a break from these words. See the final page of this text for a larger QR image.

Which grandfathers would have hated me more? The ones who first sank a flag into the soil of "Nueva España" in the 1600s, starved and overloaded with metal armor, settling and conquering and reconquering for the "glory of God"?

"¡El es dios!" ?

Or the ones who built and rebuilt and rebuilt the Socorro Mission, where I grew up praying. Did they do it (build and "pray") under a sword at first? Certainly, they worked under the weight of Catholic crosses after the first century of their servitude to the Spanish crown. By the time my Piru mestizo grandfather, Santiago, came around, they had made such pageants out of cross-bearing that he proudly carried an actual heavy wooden cross around the Mission grounds for Easter. At least one of his twelve children remembers seeing him "crucified" on it. (She seems to remember puncture wounds in his hands, too.) This was my father's father, who taught my father that the measure of his manhood was his ability to have sex with women.
No wonder my father was an unabashed bigot, especially when it came to gay and trans people. Of course, the church (conspirator with the colonial patriarchy that it has been) taught them all this. Of course, it beat self-hatred into their grandfathers and mothers. In one generation or another, they inherited the traumatic lesson/warning from those first slaughters of queer Natives: "Be like them, and you will have no place."[5]

5 Deborah A. Miranda, "Extermination of the Joyas," *GLQ* 16, nos. 1-2 (2010): 253-84. This Chumash lesbian scholar argues that the earliest and most vicious phase of Indigenous genocide was the "gendercide" committed first by colonizers against third-gender people and those found committing homosexual acts.

Must we be thankful to our ancestors for
making the sacrifices necessary to survive?
How do I thank the one who cut my heart
and my fire out from my blood? The one(s)
who choked the memory of who I can be…
so that they could breathe, live to die
another day…
Perhaps praying gratitude to them today sends
breath to them to feed (and end) the sacrifice of
yesterday… Catholicism whispers to me, telling
me that that might be forgiveness in another
form\frame…
But right now, I feel it is healing
by any means necessary.

The story I'm writing isn't your story.

But weren't your people colonized
at some point too?

The dance you do with these pages and my words is
your story

beginning.

What will you let die?
Whom will you let die?
How much will you let die?

Re-visión

I have no knowledge of the origins of the dances of my ancestral tribes (not even the ones hailing from Europe). So, you might think I have nothing to say here.

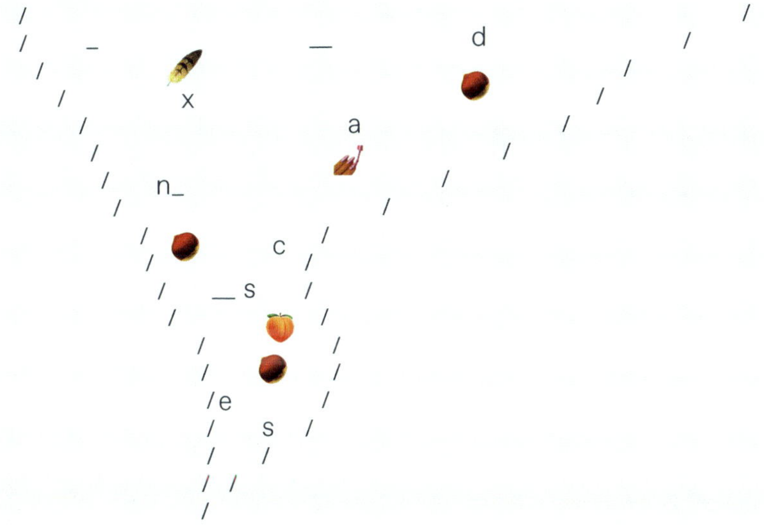

“The truth is the Ghost Dance did not end with the murder of Big Foot and one hundred and forty-four Ghost Dance worshippers at Wounded Knee. The Ghost Dance has never ended, it has continued, and the people have never stopped dancing; they may call it by other names, but when they dance, their hearts are reunited with the spirits of beloved ancestors and the loved ones recently lost in the struggle.

Throughout the Americas, from Chile to Canada, the people have never stopped dancing; as the living dance, they are joined again with all our ancestors before them, who cry out, who demand justice, and who call the people to take back the Americas!"
—Leslie Marmon Silko, *Almanac of the Dead*[6]

(An ending)

6 Leslie Marmon Silko, *Almanac of the Dead: A Novel* (New York: Simon and Schuster, 1991), 724.

Storm of Flame

I first really and fully danced before the storms that would hit my family farm in El Paso, Texas. What people think of as the calm before the storm was, for me, numinous. The electricity in the air was irresistible, charging my skin with a taut heat, spawning waves of goosebumps. My breath became shallow as my ears and eyes cast their attention outward, beyond the adobe bricks of our hundred-year-old home, beyond the farm's perimeter to the arriving clouds and descending horizon. I felt pulled as if by spears of lightning within me surging outward and up. I almost had no choice but to dance. But I did so fearfully, "foolishly," while outside, trying to look around to make sure that no one would see me…

Yet, hilariously, I remember most
being in the middle of the driveway, the
most on-stage private spot around.

The storm frequently danced me; it was one
of my first teachers…
Those were the dances of a child…

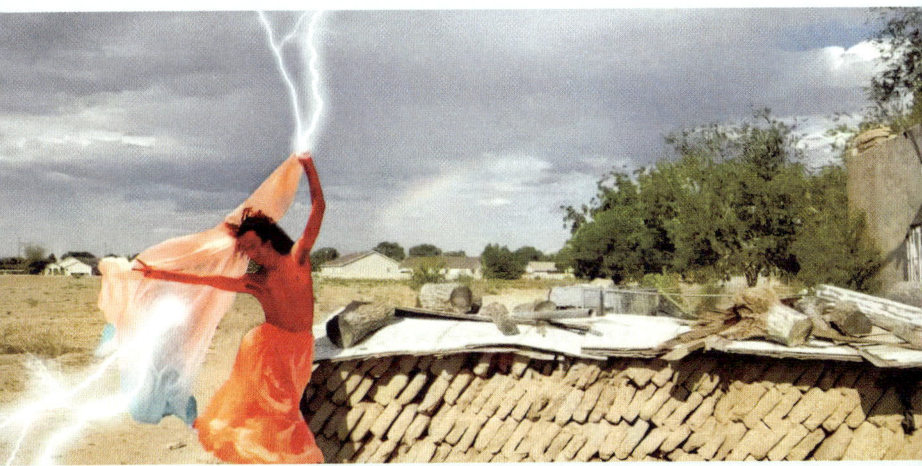

This is the beginning of a storm dance of an adult/hurt child. A score in development for a performance piece I am building. The piece will connect the violences that brought about the fires of the West Coast with those that ravage the Amazon. The stage directions for the performer are in parentheses and italicized.

Stage note: Audience sits in a black-box theater in the round. Immersive projections of a charred California landscape are visible on four sides. A nonbinary performer is present, wearing a white, semitransparent, ankle-length skirt. Depending on their level of dysphoria that day and their willingness to be bare-chested before the audience, they may wear a nude bra that matches their olive complexion.

"You know, I have a shameless confession,

soy sinverguenza.

I really enjoy gender-reveal parties!
Babies are fucking adorable, and everyone gets so excited imagining what the little guy or girl will be. Has anyone here had a gender-reveal party?
Oh, c'mon?!
Is anyone going to one? Has anyone gone to one?"
(listen for audience response)

(interrupting, while holding a box full of ashen logs)
"—You see, the thing about babies is that we project our hopes for the future onto them.
Who doesn't want progress? Who doesn't hope for better?"
(beat)

(unpacking the box, pulling out ashen logs slowly)
"But what 'heterosexual' person hopes for a queer future? Has anyone here spent time really imagining what a queer world would even look like?
What hetero person hopes for a queer world?

How straight is the world you live in—actually?"
(shoving hand into box to pull out more ashes)
"How straight is the world, the box, you put your baby inside?"
(beginning to shake) "How hot is that world?
How insulated is the box?

How wild is the baby? How tame? How well-behaved?
How *savage*?
Don't you want a little savage?!"

Here the spoken text glitches and intermingles with recorded and distorted words, and the projection fades to footage of California mega-infernos. Through a combination of footwork and stomping, high-intensity bass pulses from subwoofers and large fans, and the visceral electricity of a thunderstorm is summoned.

Recording heard with distortion from speakers:

In 2020, the El Dorado fire in San Bernardino, California, was ignited by a firework set off during a gender-reveal party. It burned twenty-three thousand acres, destroying homes and killing a firefighter and countless more-than-human relatives.

"This world is already burning, and you with babies
are already in it...
How queer is your baby's world? *(baby voice giggles
and says "Imagine?")*
Your baby's in our world...burning...for their own...
Your babies are burning...The future is burning...
for their own..."

till Queerdom come

"The land is already ready to burn...The land
in the future will burn...
Your babies on the land in the future burning...
The land in your future burns with the babies...
Your babies in this land burn with the land...

What if to save the future we must burn yours
to the ground?"

end of score

(An ending of this book)

¡*HÍJOELA*! GOOD THING <THAT'S< NOT THE LAST PAGE, EH?!

My colleague, sometimes mentor, forever vogue father, and dear friend wrote what follows some years ago, in a time of great mental and physical sickness and intentional redirection. I read it for the first time while drafting this book. It reminds me that even though we come from radically different peoples and live radically different lives, we hold similar medicines. I'm honored to include his water offering here.

Eye of the Storm

an excerpt from and possible ending to P. Don'Té Cuauhtémoc's Choreographic Essay "Monsoon"

Stand on the chair. Speak this text.

Maybe the issue is that I am code-weaving and not code-switching. That is what I have had to think about for a while. That I speak in Indigenous languages, codes, slang, traditional Indigenous knowledge...

I write that there is a storm inside me and that it is the source of my energy, my creativity, and my intellectualism. It is my mitote, my dreaming together of my spirits, my ancestors, my legacy in genealogy that is the spiritual force inside my body. And the storm is great, shady, scary, and mysterious to those who do not understand that it is a storm. I had to listen to it, show its eye, sit in the eye, and explain it to others. Others had to listen and know that the storm can be gentle, generous, and destructive—but, too, directed and expanded. In doing this, I can be supported, and my illnesses, which are based in isolation, fear, and rejection, can be absolved. From neglect, to loving embrace, from tsunami, to flood of gentle sunlight—the storm is in me and is me.

I am not my illness, the illness is the spiritual decay of care from non-Indigenous practices. With the energy of listening and my storm, my healing can be brought forth, and so can the healing of others. In looking closely to the work of healing, the goal for me is to "sew myself together…"[7]

7 Cuauhtémoc, "Monsoon," 9-10.

Weave

Play song "Throw the Shade Away" by Electric Fields. Vogue to song, the ol' way…
This dance is best done to the east, which is the direction of sunrise and new beginnings according to the medicine-circle practice in American Indian church. Yellow colors or items should be a part of this dance.[8]

8 Ibid., 12.

(Another ending)

Dancing Ourselves into Being

. . . And then I remember

I carry a dance that reimagines the Sky Woman origin story from a queer Apache two-spirit's lens. P. Don'Té Cuauhtémoc, a mixed-ancestry Mescalero Apache, Chichimeca, and Cano, and the practitioner of Mexica dance who choreographed the dance (drawing on Mexica forms, vogue performance movement, and canonical modern dance), called it *The Boy Who Fell from the Sky*. He gifted me the dance in a (contemporary) traditional way, indicating it is mine to grow, share, reshape, and learn from.

I carry the dance and share it as a gender-fluid two-spirit, not regendering Sky Woman away from womanhood but rather sharing the imagining that she, like so many first beings, was two-spirit, fluid, and multifaceted, containing multitudes . . .

As I write this, I realize the dance invites us to contemplate Sky Woman's chaotic fall as a first life-giving dance.

The story of Sky Woman that I'm familiar with is a Haudenosaunee origin story. She digs a hole in the ground of her world until she falls through it into ours . . .

Release
down into deep bent knees, letting all your
weight buckle into your ankles;
your hands shoot upward but are dragged
down by your hips.
Everything is spiraling quickly now as your wrists,
then ankles, then elbows each take turns
pulling at your core.
You gather that core to stand, balanced briefly on
one leg, with all your other limbs out to the side,
an angular bird in flight,
then release into the fall again,
*^a cycle of 8^*

As she digs and falls, her nails gather many things, including seeds that she later shares with our world.

You land gracefully out of your bird balance, a pas de chat where your long-nailed hand claws sensuously at the air in front of you, and you notice the dirt(y) underneath (of) your nails as your hips and feet pulse to a soft one-two step. Your hip pulses around back and outward on the same side as that long-nailed hand, and the step takes you in a promenade around the space, as close to your audience as feels right, but safe, but insistent—
seduce them,
only for this moment
(they may fight or flee the next).
As if to say "I pull you toward this offering...
You know you want it...
Your ancestors wanted it before you..."

As you flick your nails outward as if to scatter glittery seeds, look at everyone present, reminding them they are here.

This dance in this time of two-spirit revisibilization offers seeds of possibility to all, especially Indigenous folks ready to decolonize gender and sexuality in their cultures.

With a lofted, powerful arm carriage, I,
great bird
swoop in circles, gazing upon the land beneath me,

drop down into it, connecting sky and earth,
then, rolling on the ground to gather strength, I push
up with the earth.

\+

Sending blessings in four directions
from their center,
spirals that dizzy me. Wary in this new world,
newness spirals through me into it.

\+

Shoulders collapse forward, snapping my spine over and
shut out
from my two-spirit center of the four directions.
a blessing
ripped from the world, caught mid inhale
a blessing
lodged
spine-deep frozen
as my body spasms to spiral it out
intoxicated pandemic inhaled
hardest in the club
spine blood snaps

I fall again

quick to bless again

+

at last with vogue hands spiraling a clap
the blessing's out

+

and close in balanced flight—
fallen?

Zoom In

The Boy Who Fell from the Sky offers reflections of queer self-formation, being, and becoming that LGBTQ2S++ Natives can hold onto. Like so many expressions of two-spirit thriving and resilience, it is a seed, a packet of encoded instructions that traces back to our ancient origins. Nourishing and promising life in the future... if cared for.

I hold it in as traditional a way as I
know. Still I try to pray through it.
Still I try to attend to what it will offer
each day that I practice it.

It is a beginning.

It is two-spirit history in the making.

(Another ending)

Dear Reader,

This offering is an invitation for you to see what I've seen, a path through some of the influences and encounters that have helped form my views on dance. I pull from an atmospheric reference cloud, an archival buffet, a feast laid out in glorious bounty to be eaten by desirous mouths from the hand; I pull from the street, from videos I've happened upon on the internet, memories I can barely remember, dances I've seen and embodied. These moments have shaped and framed who I am, what I look for in the world, and how I define my life's devotion to dance. Like journal pages or image bursts in space and time, I hope these fragments read to you like a dance in verse.

My chronology and geography are flexible. The dates in the footnotes that mark these encounters in time are noted by the year I experienced them and not necessarily by the year that they were created, invented, or born, though at times the dates are marked by their own time line, not mine.

People and places shape us, and these are some of the encounters that have shaped me, and maybe some of these have also shaped you.

Lydia Okrent flies across the stage in the arms of Strauss Bourque-LaFrance.[1]

1 *ODE, DIV III concert* (2006), choreographed by Strauss Bourque-LaFrance for a shared evening with Sher Ahmad and Mariana Valencia, Hampshire College, Amherst, Massachusetts.

The curtain rises to reveal a sea
of empty red theater seats.
The dancers balance on one leg.
Their opposite legs and torsos
are extended flat, creating the illusion
that they're floating.[2]

2 *Everyone* (2007), choreographed by Miguel Gutierrez, Abrons Art Center, New York, copresented with Danspace Project, New York.

She voraciously eats a whole banana
like a beaver munching wood.
She tosses the banana peel onto
the stage floor, and we laugh about
the potential of her slipping on it.[3]

3 *ha: a solo* (2011), choreographed by Adrienne Truscott, Danspace Project, New York.

"I hate to brag, y'all, but I've been
raped twice."[4]

4 *Asking for It: A One-Lady Rape about Comedy Starring Her Pussy and Little Else!* (2013), choreographed by Adrienne Truscott, The Creek & The Cave, Long Island City, New York.

Gillian Walsh sits calmly at a table,
eating chunks of meat that she
plucks from a rotisserie chicken.
I want to eat the chicken, too.
An endless pot of tea flows into
a teacup that never overflows.
I want to know how this is possible.
Adrienne Truscott dances with
headphones on, blowing bubbles
with her gum. I want to know what
music she is listening to. I want
to know if the gum has any flavor left.
Two Latino carpenters build a
house frame and perform their labor.
Labor, labor, labor.[5]

5 *...Too Freedom...* (2012), choreographed by Adrienne Truscott, the Kitchen, New York.

A loud clamor behind a closed door goes on for an absurd amount of time. It's hilarious because David Neumann is in there.[6]

Melissa McCarthy exits her car in slow motion with a paper bag on her head, a balm for soothing what's rough.[7]

Ronan and Katie dance in a plaza.[8]

An intoxicated man falls all over everything in the store of a gas station with a six-pack in hand. We laugh at this video as it plays on a computer; we hold some sadness behind the laughter because we know that the man won't remember what his body has done—which is an awful feeling—yet he's made such a brilliant dance of it all.[9]

The blood of three chickens is sprinkled on the floor as an offering. The sacrificial pig is split lengthwise; one half hangs at the north entrance, the other half at the south entrance. The carcass blood collects in gourds below. The sea is at the east entrance, which is left open to let in the ancestors. West is the enclosed altar.[10]

6 *genesis, no!* (2008 remount), choreographed by Adrienne Truscott, Dance Theater Workshop, New York. Premiered 2007 at Performance Space 122, New York.

7 *Tammy*, directed by Ben Falcone (Burbank, CA: Warner Brothers, 2014).

8 *Love on the Spectrum*, season 2, directed by Cian O'Clery (Sydney: Australian Broadcasting Corporation, 2021).

9 "Hillarious Intoxicated Drunk Guy Falling All Over Everything in a Gas Station Must See," video posted by Epic Failers on YouTube, August 28, 2015, https://www.youtube.com/watch?v=ZPIV3O87TmA.

10 Dugu ritual, second ceremony, Garifuna sacred dance, Barranco, Belize, 2005.

I thank the woman next to me for catching me while I was out; I must have briefly lost consciousness.[11]

11 Dugu ritual, first ceremony, Garifuna sacred dance, Barranco, Belize, 2005.

Dance Muppets, contemporary dance Fraggles:

1

A dancer creeps across the altar of the Judson Church. The lights are bright, and she's committed to an odd, satisfyingly frontal, and sagittal movement. I wonder how her flat paper costume stays stuck to her body.[12]

2

Kyli Kleven, Tess Dworman, and Caitlin Marz are in a pile of their own bodies and brown hair. They move in a slippery yet suctional way.[13]

3

luciana achugar navigates the path of a light beam and wears a dark hooded cape and sings a song I know from my childhood. "Sana sana colita de rana…si no sanas hoy…sanarás mañana."[14]

4

Larissa Velez-Jackson frantically mutters something while staying close to the wall at stage right. I think, *Oh, this is dance.*[15]

The stage is empty, and the lighting design is serving doom or loss, the feeling of standing at the edge of an

12 *Desire Dances* (2011), choreographed by Moriah Evans, Movement Research at the Judson Church, New York.

13 *macromen* (2014), choreographed by Tess Dworman, New York Live Arts.

14 *Puro Deseo* (2010), choreographed by luciana achugar, the Kitchen, New York.

15 *Jeliza-Rose Is With Us* (2008), choreographed by Hilary Clark, the Kitchen, New York.

empty pit. A distorted voice lavishly recites, "Laptop on the crotch, let the vagina breathe." [16]

16 *Untitled* (2015), choreographed by Strauss Bourque-LaFrance, the Kitchen, New York.

My wife throws the lambskin rug high up in the air. She swiftly prances beneath it before it lands. She knows about theater; she's got some improv in her too. [17]

17 Charlotte Curtis, Brooklyn, New York, 2021.

I'm in a college-library carrel, and the TV plays a film where Ishmael Houston-Jones dances and speaks to the camera. His mom is draped over his shoulder as he enters the frame and places her upright on a chair. There's a small table next to her that holds a bowl of dye and a bowl of white eggs. She dyes the eggs as Ishmael dances beside her. He wears pants, shoes, and a tank top, all black. Her dress is white with flowers. There's a house in the background. [18]

18 *Relatives*, directed by Julie Dash, choreographed by Ishmael Houston-Jones (St. Paul, MN: Twin Cities Public Television, 1989).

I'm in a college-library carrel, and the TV plays a film where they dance in sneakers under an overpass. I yearn for the day when I can move to New York to do what they're doing. [19]

19 *Pull Your Head to the Moon . . . Stories Of Creole Women* (1992), directed by Ayoka Chenzira, created and choreographed by David Roussève.

Elizabeth Orr leaves a message on my dorm-room phone: "Hi, it's the day of your Div III; congratulations, I can't wait to see it." [20]

20 Hampshire College, Amherst, Massachusetts, 2006.

Trans Women
Queer Youth
Elder Queers
Mothers
Fathers
Brothers
Sisters
Cousins
Candy
Beer
and
Chip vendors dance in the street, under highways, in park plazas, and in the jail; yes, the jail.[21]

21 Sonideros, ethnographic study, Mexico City, 2015.

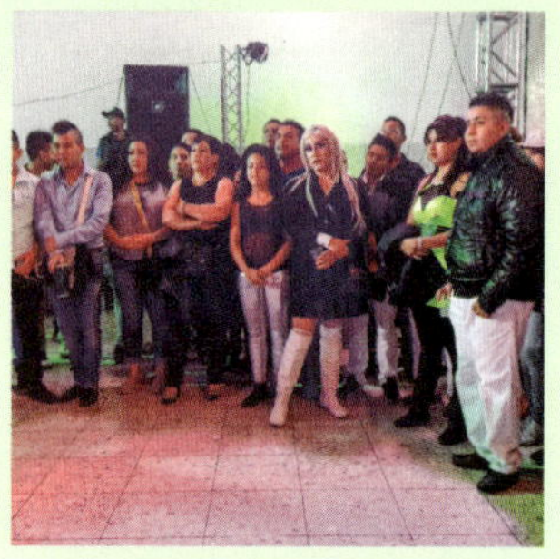

It's a dance whenever Cantinflas does anything. Everyone else just wishes they could be as good as him, and I mean everyone—Trisha, Alvin, Misha.[22]

22 Mario Fortino Alfonso Moreno Reyes (August 12, 1911–April 20, 1993), Mexican comedian, actor, and filmmaker better known as Cantinflas.

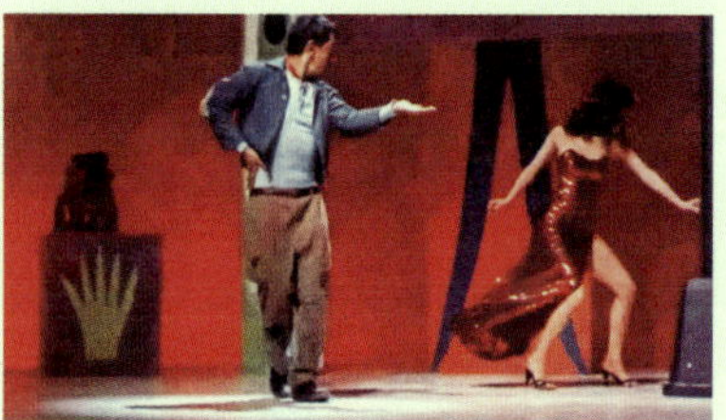

Walter Mercado speaks to us about our horoscopes. We bask in the TV glow of his queer-prophet realness.[23]

23 Walter Mercado (March 9, 1932–November 2, 2019), Puerto Rican astrologer whose predictions were broadcast by Univision television network, 1990s–2010.

La Lupe rips off her clothes while singing on television. No one sees this coming, but knowing her, we know it's possible.[24]

24 Lupe Victoria Yolí Raymond (December23,1936–February 29, 1992), Cuban entertainer better known as La Lupe.

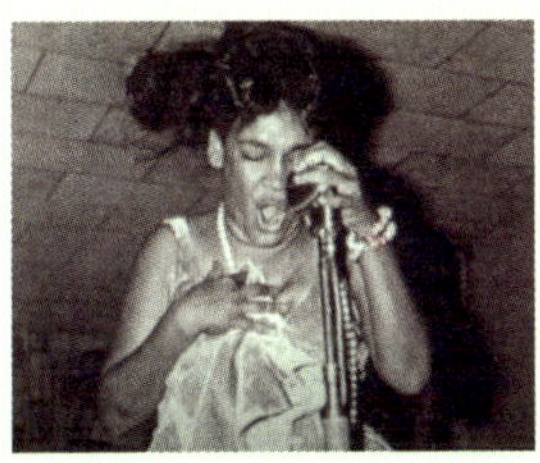

It's a dinner party where the people dance around the table to "Day-O" by Harry Belafonte. It's some sort of seance that's supposed to rid the house of the ghosts that haunt it. The food on their plates comes alive, clawlike, and grabs the people by their faces.[25]

25 *Beetlejuice* (1988), directed by Tim Burton (Los Angeles: Geffen Company, 1988).

This is how I remember it:
Bill T. Jones and Arnie Zane leap through a vast, empty space at MASS MoCA. Bill says, "A system in collapse is a system moving forward."[26]

26 This is mostly a memory that I cannot find the source of. Does this count as history? I need help finding the footage; email me at marianavalenciawork@gmail.com.

The ring shout.[27]

27 The Deep South.

The Lindy hop.[28]

28 Harlem, New York.

Tap dance.[29]

29 William Henry Lane (c. 1825–c. 1852–53), Black American dancer better known as Master Juba.

Slam dunks.[30]

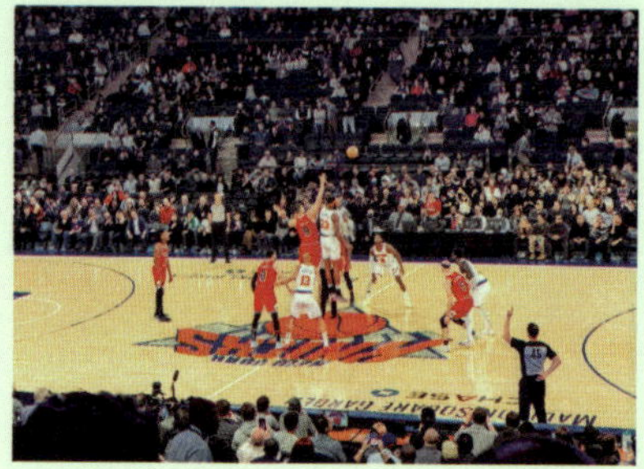

30 Michael Jordan, basketball player for the Chicago Bulls during my childhood. And Bulls vs. Knicks, Madison Square Garden, New York, my first time at a basketball game, March 2022.

Our bodies dance pressed together at the party, where we hold our drinks above the crowd so that we don't spill, but there's spilling anyway. We whisper-shout into one another's ears to flirt. We're as loud and as young as we'll ever be.[31]

31 Prescott House, Hampshire College, Amherst, Massachusetts, 2002–6.

"Pussy."[32]

32 *Bronx Gothic* (2014), choreographed by Okwui Okpokwasili, Danspace Project, New York.

niv Acosta and another performer sing in an empty bathtub that's set up in the middle of a loft in Bushwick, Brooklyn.[33]

33 Aunts Is Dance, New York, an organization that supports the development of current, present, and contemporary dancing through events and parties, 2005-ish.

Yakez performs for the first time in a loft in Bushwick, Brooklyn. Larissa says something about "coming out of her mama."[34]

34 Aunts Is Dance, New York, 2011-ish.

The long, long limbs of Kennis Hawkins and Will Rawls dancing together.[35]

35 New York, early 2000s.

Talking about making dance with Katie Workum, Mina Nishimura, and Catherine Galasso.[36]

36 Chez Bushwick Artist-in-Residence (AIR) program, Brooklyn, New York, 2013.

Addys Gonzalez[37]

37 The dancer and my friend, New York, early 2000s–present.

Eleanor Hullihan is in a red leotard and sneakers. She runs forever. Non Griffiths is in a contortion and all in white. Her arms and legs in a grab.[38]

38 *Devotion* (2011), choreographed by Sarah Michelson, the Kitchen, New York.

Strauss Bourque-LaFrance[39]

39 The dancer and my friend, Western Massachusetts, Philadelphia, Los Angeles, and New York, 2002–present.

I empty my apartment and invite my friends to see a dance I've made where 33 mm slide collages play on a wall and my costume is made of plastic tarp. I've hung plastic sculptures from the ceiling. We end with a parade—a circular path through my railroad apartment and hallway. My best friend from childhood, Keely Johnson, is here. I record the event and use the video as a work sample to book future gigs. I have so much hope for this work.[40]

40 *FORT* (2007), choreographed by Mariana Valencia, Brooklyn, New York.

The dancers climb the theater walls and beat them in percussive splendor. The surfaces begin to dent, and it's thrilling to see it happen. They're informing The Institution.[41]

41 *OTRO TEATRO* (2014), choreographed by luciana achugar, New York Live Arts.

His arms reach forward as he planks backward to the floor; he's full of tension as the spiritual "I Wanna Be Ready" roars from the chorus singers.[42]

42 *Revelations* (1960), choreographed by Alvin Ailey, premiered at Kaufman Concert Hall, 92nd Street Y, New York.

It's the lockdown, and I'm drinking my morning coffee. The dance I'm watching on my computer is danced on a rooftop. And I can't tell if this footage is captured against a sunrise or a sunset, but the sky's in an orangey-pink mood. The dancer moves up and down the slope of the roof, from one side to the other and almost to the edge.[43]

43 Benjamin Akio Kimitch dancing on a New York rooftop, *AUNTS WPA: micro stimulus*, Aunts Is Dance Instagram Live program, March 21, 2020.

Erin Markey speaks in gibberish, and I understand every word![44]

44 *Work-in-progress* (2013–15), created by Erin Markey, Brooklyn Arts Exchange, Brooklyn, New York.

Lydia Okrent[45]

45 The dancer and my friend, Western Massachusetts, Philadelphia, and New York, 2002–present.

Tai and Cher enter a house party; Cher kneels on one knee while holding Tai's hand. Tai sensually walks around Cher, lets go of her hand, and shakes her breasts at the camera. I want to be her, and I'm in love with her.[46]

46 *Clueless*, directed by Amy Heckerling (Los Angeles: Paramount Pictures, 1995).

We're gazing into the Grecian night sky, and we both see the same shooting star.[47]

47 Santorini, Greece, July 2019.

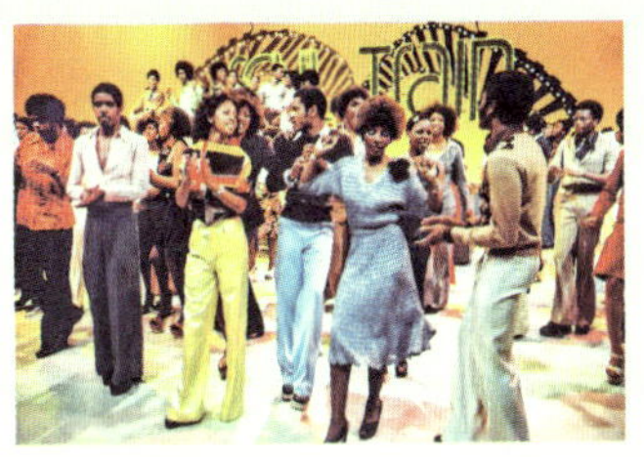

I begin my dance career in the same television studio *Soul Train* began in in Chicago.[48]

48 *Soul Train*, aired 1971–2006.

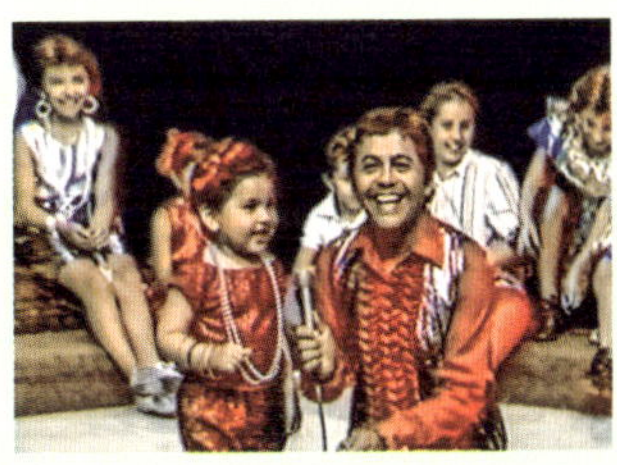

I'm dancing in the television studio. My mom and nanny stand camera-side. The "ON AIR" light glows over the door to the greenroom as the cameraperson rolls tape.[49]

49 El Club Del Niño, television show hosted by Palomo on channel 26 (WGBO), Chicago, 1980s.

Jacklean prefers the pronouns *we* and *us*.[50]

50 *Jacklean (The Future)*, created by Lydia Okrent and Mariana Valencia on the floor of a studio at Dance Theater Workshop, New York, 2014.

The bags are all different types, and they speak to her. They just sit there on the stage floor, and words come out of them. These are bags. No one has ever seen or made a performance like this.[51]

51 *Bags* (2007), created by Dynasty Handbags (Jibz Cameron), Dance Theater Workshop, New York.

Four dancers spiral to the earth, descending from a tall, tall pole. I'm eating spicy peanuts topped with lime juice from a plastic baggie—the most perfect snack. My fingers are stained red from the chile on the peanuts, which is also the color of the dancers' pants. The dancers' torsos are tied to ropes that suspend them upside down in a unison spiral motion. 52

52 Los Voladores de Papantla, performing La Danza de los Voladores, Museo Nacional de Antropología, Mexico City, 2015.

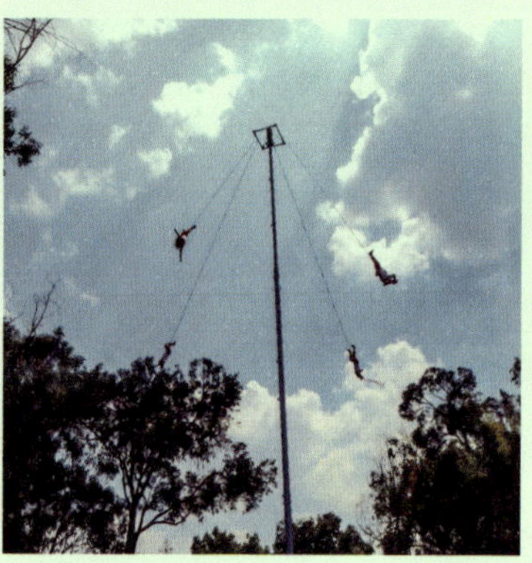

My grown-ups and I take turns dancing with my grandmother at her ninetieth birthday party. 53

53 Abuelita's ninetieth birthday party, Chicago, 2021.

Amelia Bande's singing voice plucks its way through the party; she plays a mini-keyboard and sings about everyday moments with a not-so-everyday delivery. 54

54 W.A.G.E. RAGE, New York, 2018; BOFFO Fire Island Performance Festival, Fire Island Pines, New York, 2018; Instagram Live, 2021.

I thank all the goddesses when Kathy Kaufmann takes the lead at tech. 55

55 Danspace Project, New York, 2017; American Realness, New York, 2018; the Chocolate Theater, Long Island City, New York, 2019; Performance Space New York, 2020; Fringe Festival, Philadelphia, 2021; Abrons Arts Center, New York, 2022.

I want to touch Aretha Aoki's legs because they make me think of moles—the mammal kind, not the skin kind. She's full of gravity and face down on the floor; her leggings are black velour.[56]

56 *Las Gravitas* (2013), choreographed by Aretha Aoki, Danspace Project, New York.

Joey Kipp's in a nun's habit and startles a person in the audience with an unexpected "boo."[57]

57 *Sister Jean Ra Horror* (2015), choreographed by Joey Kipp, Roulette, Brooklyn, New York.

I bike through an urban prairie and see a grouping of nonperishable foods on a table; a sign reads "free store." I then pass a partially decomposed cat carcass.[58]

58 AUNTS X Detroit Residency, organized by Aunts Is Dance, 2016.

A baby crawls along the bottom step of a bank that towers over her. Her mother works at a stand selling combs, phone chargers, barrettes, and women's underwear.[59]

59 Colonia Roma, Mexico City, 2015.

A taco truck down the block has a bundle of gray next to it. The bundle's moving; she's a baby. Her clothes are soiled gray, and she's learning to crawl on top of a piece of cardboard on the sidewalk.[60]

60 Coyoacán, Mexico City, 2015.

Stanley Love looks at me and tells me that I'm a brilliant child and that there's a brilliant glow coming out of me. I've only been in New York a few years, and his blessing makes New York feel like home. Stanley Love was our blessing.[61]

61 Dancer and choreographer Stanley Love (March 17, 1970–August 22, 2019) at *I believe in you*, organized by Aunts Is Dance, the Event Center, Brooklyn, 2008.

Tess Dworman looks into the distance while swinging a tote bag around. That stare, that tote bag.[62]

62 *Legendary Children* (2011), choreographed by Tess Dworman, Brazil Studio, Brooklyn.

Tingying Ma takes us on a ride. It's about a bento box, it's about seeing her walk from a bird's-eye view, and it's about someone's birthday. This is a dance.[63]

63 *A Child Retires* (2019), choreographed by Tess Dworman, the Chocolate Factory Theater, Long Island City, New York.

Lauren Bakst sings a ska song into a mic; she's perfectly embodied and skews awkward-but-completely-fine-with-it. A certain "fuck you" emanates from her. I'm infected by the irreverent vibe she's serving.[64]

64 *More Problems with Form* (2019), choreographed by Lauren Bakst, the Chocolate Factory Theater, Long Island City, New York.

Lydia Okrent starts crying—and quickly switches to a fit of jumping, like a possessed frog or maybe a killer. She's unrecognizable to me; I'm bewildered as tears plop onto the program in my hand.[65]

65 *Configure* (2018), choreographed by Moriah Evans, the Kitchen, New York.

I video-chat on my phone device with mayfield brooks about writing this book.[66]

66 Video chat, 2021.

She says, "Everything you have is yours?" into a lavalier mic on her head that makes her voice crisp like a public-radio broadcast. Her shirt is neatly tucked into her sensible jeans; she dances and tells us where the dances come from.[67]

67 *Everything You Have Is Yours?* (2017), choreographed by Hadar Ahuvia, Brooklyn Studios for Dance, Brooklyn, New York.

Stuffed animals are thrown at Levi Gonzalez from the audience. In another section, he puts down a thin plastic sheet and performs a "tap dance."[68]

68 *Clusterfuck* (2007), choreographed by Levi Gonzalez, Dance Theater Workshop, New York.

Mina Nishimura[69]

69 The dancer and my friend, New York, early 2000–present.

Maria Hassabi stretches and folds herself in many directions, and the pillars onstage frame her just right.[70]

70 *Solo* and *SoloShow* (both 2009), choreographed by Maria Hassabi, Performance Space 122, New York.

I'm on Second Avenue waiting to enter a dance show by robbinschilds (Sonya and Layla) and I'm giddy about it because everyone here might be queer. During the performance, a video plays in which Sonya and Layla dance against a rocky landscape. During the performance, a duet structure and clothing items make a rainbow tableau.[71]

71 *C.L.U.E.(color location ultimate experience)* (2007), choreographed by robbinschilds (Sonya Robbins and Layla Childs), Performance Space 122, New York.

Ali Rosa-Salas sits at a table on the porch of the farmhouse where we've just met. I have the feeling we're going to know each other for a long time.[72]

72 *Camp* (2015), residency organized by Aunts Is Dance, Mount Tremper Arts, Mount Tremper, New York.

I'm on a Zoom call with Ali, and Mikhail Baryshnikov (Misha) enters. It's pretty cool.[73]

73 Zoom video conference, 2021.

Sometimes, the first time you see someone, you just know you'll keep trying to see them again.

Julie Tolentino leads us in her practice called the Pressure, in which two or more people press into each other, at times partially, at times as a wrapping of bodies, a practice of intention and physical impression. Lift the ones who need lifting. Lift up through gravity. The gravity is in each of us.[74]

74 *Marking the Occasion* (2019), residency organized by Jaime Shearn Coan and Tara Aisha Willis, Mount Tremper Arts, Mount Tremper, New York.

"Desert Water."
"What?"
"Exactly…"[75]

75 *Desert Water*, invented by Elsa Brown, Lydia Okrent, and Mariana Valencia, Joshua Tree, California, 2014.

Levi and I eat a delicious (and free) nothing-omelet for breakfast every morning.[76]

76 Global Practice Sharing Residency, Serbia and Macedonia, 2016.

I'm at my friend's eleventh birthday party at the roller rink, and "Follow Me" by Aly-Us starts playing. In a speedy fit of gorgeousness and bliss, Matan Levi skates by me while unbuttoning his shirt. My hormones are destroyed by what he's just done.[77]

77 Rainbow Roller Skate, Chicago, 1995.

"Go have a go,
Go have a go,
Go get them there and bring
them down."[78]

78 *Folk Incest* (2018), choreographed by Juliana F. May, Abrons Arts Center, New York.

Josephine Baker[79]

79 American-born French entertainer (June 3, 1906–April 12, 1975).

My mom dances to disco music in the living room (eyes closed). She's in the slow-motion energy of a memory, under the shimmer of a disco ball, surrounded by her activist comrades and gay friends.[80]

80 My mother, Ileana Valencia, Chicago, Illinois, 1984–present.

It's Wednesday night at Crazy Legs Skate Club; if you know, you know.[81]

81 Crazy Legs Skate Club, Brooklyn, New York, 2000s.

Lupe and I are at the Café Tacvba concert; the mosh pit, the shoving, the energy.[82]

82 Café Tacvba concert with Guadalupe Rosales, Manhattan Center, New York, 2013.

Lupe and I are at the Juan Gabriel concert, making our mothers' dreams come true at Madison Square Garden. He's so gay, we're so gay, the audience is so Brown, everyone is singing *con amor*.[83]

83 Juan Gabriel concert with Guadalupe Rosales, Madison Square Garden, New York, 2014.

The song changes, and so does their mood; it's a melancholy reverence.
The grown-ups trickle onto the dance floor, and the dancing happens side by side; no touching.
Step, light tap;
step, light tap.
The men hold their hands behind their backs; the women hold their skirts out slightly. They're transported to someplace I don't know, but they're all there, and I've seen them go there before. Party after party, decade after decade, their bodies remember this dance and go back to a time before there was time.[84]

84 My grown-ups dance the Guatemalan Son of the Mayan People, beginning of time–present.

I search the radio stations on my boom box to find the best house song to dance to. I find a good one and start to get down. My Polish cousin Monika watches me and tries dancing like me. I'm aware that I'm teaching her something. I'm aware that I'm dancing for myself in front of her. I'm eight, she's sixteen.[85]

85 My cousin Monika learns how to dance to house music by watching me dance to house music, Chicago, 1993.

I drink a martini and eat a burger at Julius' bar before or after Monday Night at Judson.
OR
I schlep around town all day, and I just need a place to rest, charge my phone, be gay, eat, drink, and use the bathroom, so I go to Julius'.
OR
I leave Neil Greenberg's show at Greene Naftali and go to celebrate my day at Julius', where I drink tequila and soda and eat a burger. It's a crying-in-public sort of day as I trot around Manhattan for the first time and ride the train for the first time, too. There's a pandemic. Somehow, I'm still here.[86]

86 Julius', New York, 2006–present.

The man on the G train who sings "Baby Can I Hold You" by Tracy Chapman just got on, and his performance makes whatever's going to happen today fine.[87]

87 G-train performer, Brooklyn, New York, early 2000s.

Lupe and I walk each other home from Bushwick to Crown Heights. It's not a durational dance, but it could be a durational dance. [88]

88 My friend the artist Guadalupe Rosales, Brooklyn, New York, 2013.

Jazmin and Jezenia DJ the last dance party I attend before the pandemic hits NYC. The following occurs: "Oye Mi Amor" by Maná comes on, and the white people step aside as all the Brown people rush to the center of the dance floor, and we lose our minds dancing. We dance for ourselves in front of them. Soon after, "La Ingrata" by Café Tacvba plays, and it happens again! The white people step aside as all the Brown people rush to the center of the dance floor, and we lose our minds dancing. We dance for ourselves in front of them. Jenny Schlenzka joins us for both songs; she somehow knows what we know. [89]

89 End-of-season dance party, DJed by Jazmin and Jezenia Romero, Performance Space New York, 2020.

It's such a big hug. First, the pressure of Geo's hug cracks my bones, and then it knocks out all my breath, and then the lost breath becomes a smile, and then the laughter starts, and then the rocking begins. Geo rocks and rocks my limp body, and it feels never-ending, and it's something I can't give back with the same intensity because Geo's hugged all the strength out of me, but it feels so nice. [90]

90 My friend the artist Geo Wyex's hug, New York, 2006–present.

No Total: Elizabeth Orr, Jordan Lord, Joey Teeling, Emma Hedditch, and I lift one another up in an action we call "Bernie." The action is to take turns lifting one body at a time: Joey, Orr, Em, Jordan, Mariana. We each get a turn; we get to lift and be lifted.[91]

91 No Total reading group, Artists Space, New York, 2012–15.

We invite Fred Moten to breakfast at Artists Space Books & Talks. We're so excited about meeting Fred, and we cannot wait to ask him questions and offer him pastries, coffee, and fruits. Our secret name for the gathering is "Fred Moten Christmas."[92]

92 No Total reading group, Artists Space, New York, April 13, 2013.

I read the *Popol Vuh* for the first time, and I finally understand what a creation story can be. It can be about the trial and error of the gods, about making the perfect human after many attempts; it can be told by multiple voices; and it can teach us how to "shape and frame" ourselves and the world we tirelessly try to draw meaning from.[93]

93 *Popol Vuh*, trans. Michael Bazzett (Minneapolis: Milkweed Editions, 2018).

The grown-ups gather to do the dance-party thing where their bodies bliss together. The occasion doesn't matter; they arrive at the occasion; their arrival is a movement, and the movement is ongoing. Communion through exhaustion; hands touching, legs crossing, marking time here and here and here.

They embrace, gaze into one another's eyes,
and release loud sighs that signal that
tonight, everyone's gonna be all right. It's a
full-body good: nice clothes, perfumed skin,
hair's just right, lipstick's bright, toothy
smiles all around. If the record's tight, they
jump straight up to get down; if the record's
tight, they go inward in a prayer kind of vibe.
A baby sits on the carpet, and the grown-
ups look at her with love eyes. The music
from the speakers rattles the rug, and the
room is filled with everyone she knows.
The grown-ups pick her up tenderly and
rock her in the movement's hold. Heads
resting gently close, swaying to and fro.
And when they put her back down, she
claps at them, and they clap back; everyone
is clapping; the room is filled with clapping.
The children come in every size.
They run, pop balloons, laugh, and play.
They eat rice off clumsy paper plates.
They pour soda into party cups, stain
their fancy clothes, and politely ask the
grown-ups if they know when the cake
will be served.
At the party, the children help one another
get around. The big ones help the little
ones when they need a little cuddle.
They also pick on one another, as siblings
do. They hiss and chuckle through age-old
teases—growing pains, marking-space
kind of teases.
The children play in rooms with perfectly
made beds that hold piles of coats;

they open drawers filled with shades of
lipstick; they hide in closets that take them
into wild, imaginary places. The children
slurp up the party cheer that the grown-ups
put down; they clap their hands to the
music, and the grown-ups clap back. Witty
little dancers, cute as hell, their audience is
captive, bound by a primordial connection,
the feeling of belonging to the earth.
Everybody's clapping, everybody's proud.
Everybody's clapping, everybody's proud.
Everybody's clapping, everybody's proud.
Everybody's clapping, everybody's proud.
One of the younger grown-ups, Estrellita,
who's always busy dancing, has the
brightest, blackest eyes. And she doesn't
need a partner; her leg muscles stretch and
pulse and give and take, and the heels on
her feet smash the carpet. Estrellita's
dressed and equally bare. Like the saints at
church, she shows her body through the
drape of her garb, the kind where the drape
that covers her nakedness only accentuates
her nipple or her knee—it's like that,
Estrellita is dressed and equally bare.
In the room, there are also Lola, Lencha,
Panchi, Tito, Juanita, José, Francisco,
Bianca and Blanca, Reyna, Doris,
Roland, Susana, Pati, both Rosas,
Oscar, Raúl, Ana, Paula, Abril, Chucho,
Ricardo, Maximiliano, Renato, La Leti,
Don Marcelo, Doña Maritza, La Juli,
Esperanza, Carlos, Emiliano, Armando, Julio,
Cilda, María and Mariela, Doña Concha

and Doña Laurita and Doña Marí, Carmelita,
Lidia, Julián, Andres, Roberto, Manuelito,
Armandito, Giselle, Jazmina, Sylvia, Arcoiris,
Oro and Pilar, Evelyn, Joana, Marimar,
La Sirena, Marcos, Charito, La Chiquis,
El Negro, La Blanca, La Gorda, La Flaca,
and El Serio.
All week long, the grown-ups work
and work and work.
Day shifts and night shifts and
sometimes even both.
The grown-ups build machine parts
in factories, towel-dry at the car wash,
process chicken on conveyor belts,
scrub dishes downtown,
mow lawns in the suburbs,
clean floors at the plant,
raise white people's babies,
and tend to everything that needs tending
to with that hustle kind of diligence.
All the toilets,
all the mirrors.
They vacuum all the carpets.
All week long, they pick up,
clean up,
build up,
dry up,
mow, rock, pluck, wipe, and scrub,
day after day after day after day.
So today, they deserve this party. It's a
bridge to survival, a dance, a gathering,
a physical transcendence: communion
through exhaustion that helps them
face the week ahead. [94]

94 My grown-ups, Chicago, 1980s–present.

DANCE FORMS

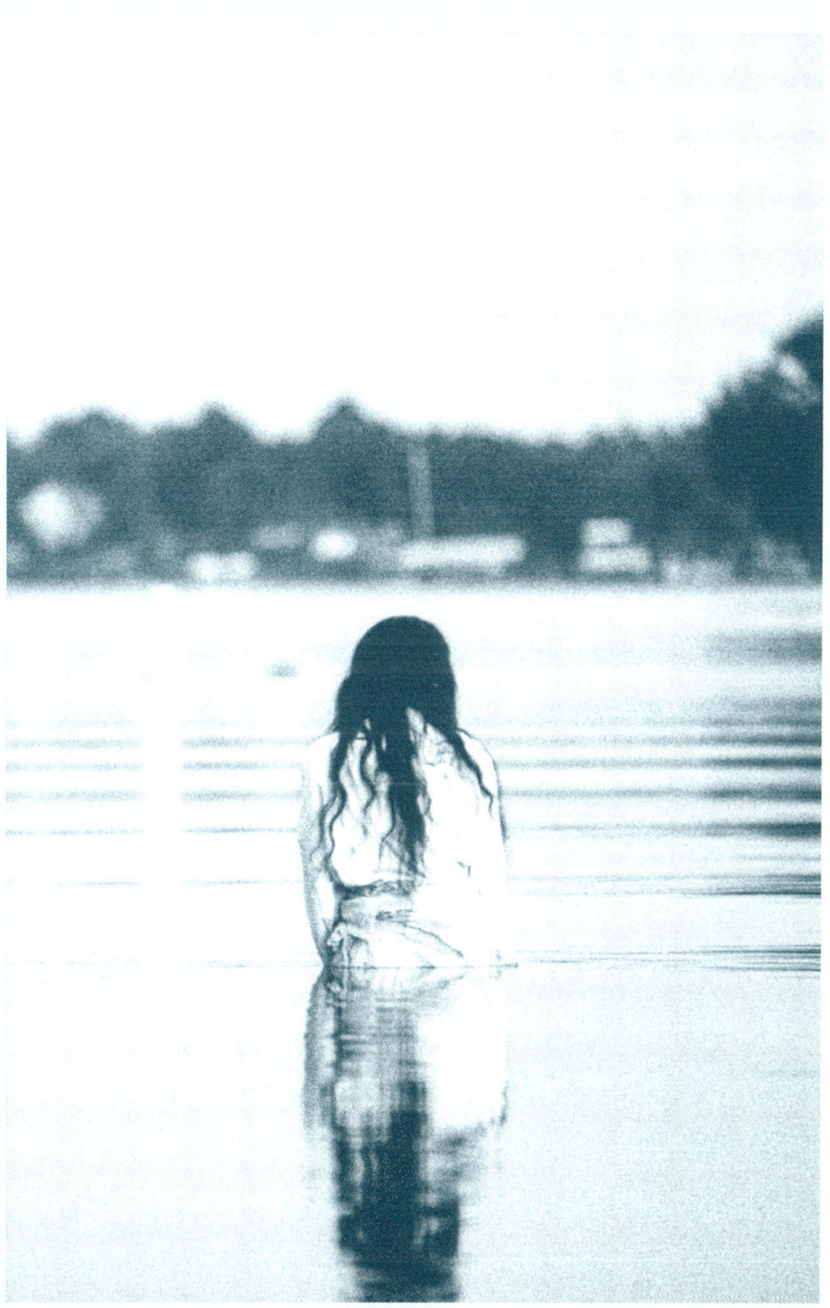

Time carries bodies
ancient bodies

Time is not even,
quiet,
or patient

Fragile

We are hurt
We hurt

Time swallows time
Time is naked

She dances to linger in that nakedness

Dance
An abundance of cries and breaths.
Bodies, lives, and movements

In 1995, Koma and I made an outdoor piece titled *River*. Over the next several years, we performed the piece *in* many rivers. The audience sat on the riverbanks. We appeared from upstream, holding onto driftwood that carried us down the river. During the performance, we moved downstream, lingering here and there, only to eventually float away into the darkness until no one could see us anymore.

Clinging to a rock, I marveled at how much water the river carries. It has done so since before I was born and will continue long after I die. The force of water pushes us. I open my pores. We are details, a small part of the whole that collects, streams, and transports to the unknown.

Accepting the flow is humbling. Taking it all in is tempting. But sometimes I resist. My choice is not only about what I take in but also about what I will not, not all the time.

I wrote letters to those who have danced and died. Each stream had come into my body, including that of Dore Hoyer, whom I have not even met. I had little dance training. But I have been inspired by certain dance artists long before me. I have written letters to them so I can remember them vividly and share these episodes with you.

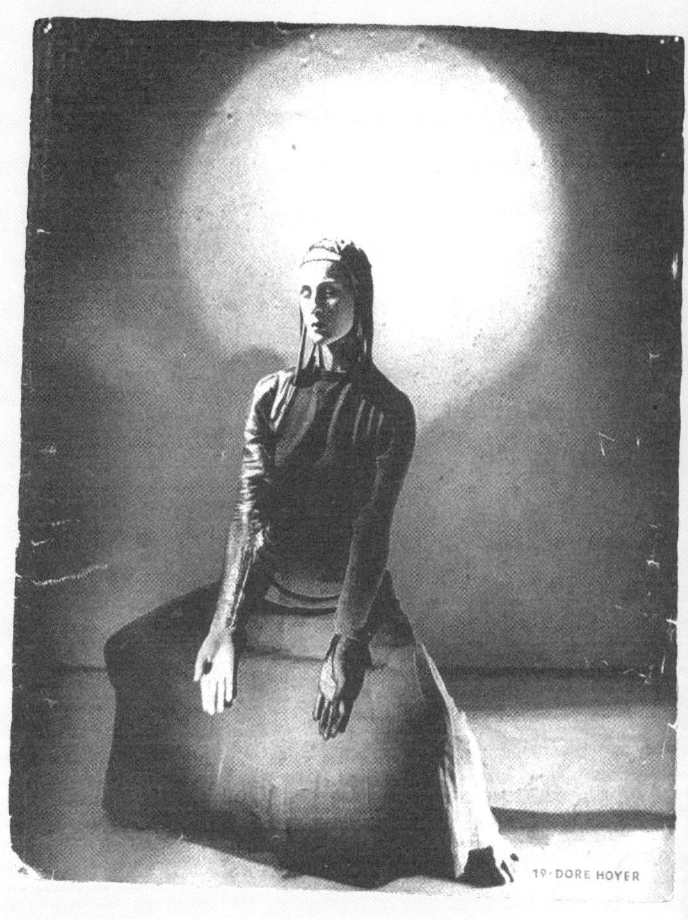

Dore Hoyer, *Tanz der erhabenen Trauer* (*Dance of the Wonderous Sorrow*) from the cycle *Der große Gesang* (*The Great Song*), 1948

Dear Dore,

I never met you.

I saw your photo in a small dance archive collection in Tokyo in 1972. I did not know who you were. I had just turned twenty. At the time, I barely knew dance history or dance artists, except several in Japan. So Koma and I went to a research room on the third floor of a concert hall in Tokyo. That is where I came across your photo, which captivated me. You are still, but I feel a strong sense of movement in your resolve. You are grounded. You are not trying to be impressive, which, in turn, impressed me. You have a quest. From this picture, I could not imagine your voice or your words. That stirred a new appetite in me. I was exhausted by words and arguments.

You are centered.

I tried your posture, staying there for as long as I could.

My teacher Kazuo Ohno was genuine and extraordinary but a man with a family. You are alone.
A woman alone.

Koma and I left Japan without knowing where we were going. But we stayed in Germany partly because it is where you lived. In Germany, we learned more about you. Mary Wigman praised you as "Europe's last great modern dancer." Though Wigman was a giant in German neuer Tanz, I saw reviews about her performance after World War II: "No More Barefoot Dance!" Despite the German people's lack of enthusiasm for modern dance in the postwar era, you were a soloist from the Wigman School. You traveled to and performed in America and Argentina.

You played the sacrifice in *The Rite of Spring* in 1957. Was that what you wanted?

I met your close friend and executor, Frau Luley, when she produced our show in Frankfurt in 1973. At her home, she showed me volumes of your photo books. Placed on top of each other, the photo albums were piled as tall as my height.

That day, I learned you always had the circling dance in your program. Without it, you would not finish your concert. By turning and turning alone, you made your body a navel of the world—an act in defiance of those who favored a group dynamic and movements in unison.

Frau Luley also told me that despite your knee injury, you spent your savings on your last performance on December 18, 1967, at Theater des Westens, but you had only a small audience. You could not offer any more concerts physically or financially. You decided to kill yourself on December 31, 1967.

The turbulent year 1968, which changed many of our generation, was about to start, but you did not see it. I am much older now than you were when you died. I want you to know that this one photograph of you made the very young me imagine you with your commitment to dance and to be seen and your desire to transform your body into art. In your last letter, you wrote,

> *Only in dance could I communicate.*

Koma and I studied with Manja Chmiel, another strong female dancer of the Wigman School. She performed solo barefoot for hours. We owe so much to Manja for her classes and support.

I close my letter to you with a photo of a necklace that Manja gave to Koma and me. Manja got it from Mary Wigman. Wigman got it from Martha Graham. Graham got it from an Indian dancer, Manja told me. I asked her, “Which Indian? Native American or from India in Asia?” She did not know the answer. In writing this letter, I realize you brought me to Germany, to Manja, and to this gift. I imagine you in this necklace, and thank you.

Respectfully,
Eiko Otake

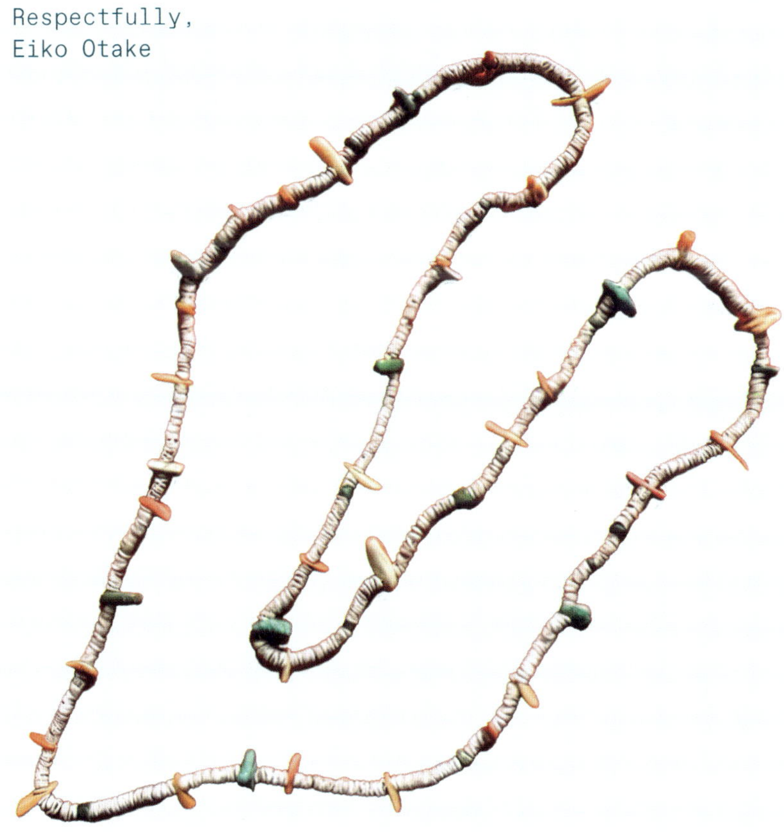

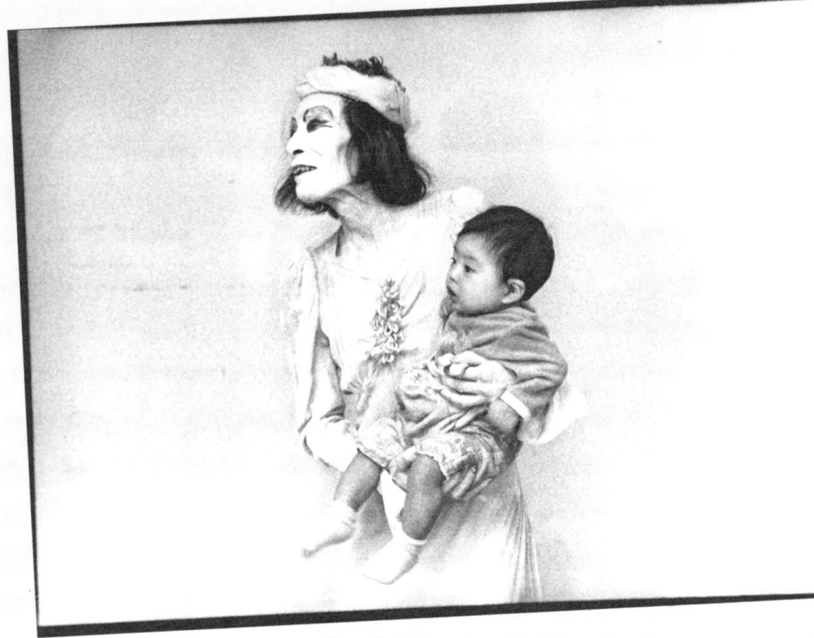

Kazuo Ohno with Yuta Otake, 1985

Dear Kazuo Ohno,

Ohno sensei, you are the only person I address as "sensei" (teacher). You were my teacher, though I never paid for your class. Being a student never suited me, but you called me your student.

Every time I saw you dance, I cried. In Munich, New York, and Japan, over and over, I was moved by a strange wind that seemed to blow from your chest, what you called a spirit, what I saw as excessive eagerness and readiness to dance. That wind swirled in the theater, and I breathed it in.

Even with dementia, you remembered me as "Eiko-live-in-New-York." During one of my visits, you took my hand to your cheek, then licked each finger and my palm for a long time. Who else could lick me so thoroughly and I would feel OK? Could your dance ever end?

When I first came to your studio in 1972, I followed the directions you gave me over the phone and was surprised to find you waiting for me at the bottom of a hill. It was a dark and cold night. After that, I walked up that slope two evenings a week to your studio for your 7:30 p.m. class. At the time, you had only a handful of students. You would say a few things, show us some pictures from time to time, and then tell us to improvise for about two hours. No other instructions before, during, or after the class. The tasks of continuously facing my own mind and feeling the limits of my imagination were so overwhelming that sometimes, upon arriving at the studio, I could not open its door. On such nights, after several minutes of hesitation, I turned around to walk down the hill in darkness. I remember that walk; it somehow became my base.

You were not yet the world-famous Kazuo Ohno. You had a day job as a school janitor. Previously, you had taught gym in the same all-girls private Christian school for decades. To everyone's surprise, you became a janitor at the regulated retirement age. You were hardly concerned with the society's hierarchy. You continued to choreograph and perform at the school's Christmas event every year, even after you became a janitor. You said you *were dancing* when you cleaned a chandelier, balancing yourself on top of a high ladder.

You were a strange teacher. We students did not relate to one another as we moved. I noticed this only when I took improvisation classes elsewhere. Dealing with others was not prohibited, but your students somehow sensed that to dance in your studio was to be alone, to face oneself.

With no air conditioner, the studio was sweaty in the summer. In the winter, with one stove and no insulation, the floor was icy cold. Though you did not ask, we were all barefoot. Somehow, we felt that was the manner. The discomfort made us move reluctantly. I sensed the music you played was for you to imagine your own dancing. I endured it.

After what felt like an unbearably long time, you called on your students to stop. No feedback was offered, but you gave us some food. We all came directly from our jobs, so when the class ended, we were all hungry. In the winter, during the class, a big pan of soup was cooking on the oil stove. Compared with classes abroad, much less was spoken in your studio. I remember the sound of others sipping the soup. Genuinely awkward.

I remember the big white chair you sat on and the large low table in front of it. I also remember several things you said.

- *Take the shortest time to enter into dance. Know you have little time to dance but behave as if you have all the time in the world.*
- *I can call an ambulance car. It could be waiting for you. Dance so you do not regret! Do not hold back.*
- *Dance with the dead.*
- *I need to dance the kind of dance that moves the spirit forward, so a body whether alive or dead will follow. Then, a body will one day disappear.*
- *When people say, "I understand your dance," I become sad. How can they, when I cannot understand my dance?*
- *While I was in my mother's body, my life was nourished at the expense of my mother's life. As she was moving to death, I was becoming.*

Sometimes, you would relay ghost stories by Lafcadio Hearn and tell us how your mother recited them at bedtime. Your mother's voice changed as she read a story, and you thought she became a ghost in the stories. And, in saying that, you became the ghost of your mother. In later years, I saw in you the joy of becoming a ghost, a dancing ghost—a ghost who is excessive and loves to be seen.

You also talked about how when you were young, you were moved by seeing a performance of Spanish dancer "La Argentina," Antonia Mercé y Luque, in 1929 at the Tokyo Imperial Theater. By seeing her only once from the third-floor balcony, you were smitten.

Soon after Koma and I came to New York in 1976, I looked her up in the Jerome Robbins Dance Division of the New York Public Library. The film footage of her performance was utterly convincing to me. Her entire body smiled as you did sometimes. She danced with a rhythmic but complex castanet sound. You danced at her grave and used in your performances a sound recording of Argentina's castanets that her relative gave you. How assertive you were in loving someone so much, a dancer you saw only once so long ago.

I filled a large envelope with photocopies of La Argentina and sent it to you. At the time, you had not publicly performed for many years. You told me how La Argentina spoke to you as the photos came out of the envelope, saying, "Kazuo, let's dance." You premiered your *Admiring La Argentina* in 1977 in Tokyo when you were seventy-one.

After that, you were unstoppable. You had your international debut at the Nancy Theater Festival in 1980. Later that year, you stopped over in New York and stayed in our apartment. You performed *Admiring La Argentina* in our friend's loft for us and other guests. When you left, I found a thank-you note with one thousand dollars in cash under the pillow on the bed you slept in. You were worried about us and thanked us for sending you La Argentina's seduction.

The following year, at the age of seventy-five, you came back to New York for your official New York debut at La MaMa and gave six performances, alternating *Admiring La Argentina* with your new piece, *My Mother*. In your body, I saw your mother. You told us you dreamed of her as a jellyfish floating on your palm. Standing ovations.

Invitations came to you from all over the world. In 1985, you were at the Joyce Theater in New York. In 1988, at the Asia Society. You came back for sold-out performances at Japan Society in 1993 and 1996.

I saw Susan Sontag run down the stairs to greet you. Allen Ginsberg happily looked through the glass door while you showered after the show. When Richard Schechner asked, "How do you calm down?" you said, "I do not wish to calm down." I was there as a translator.

You loved cameras. Even for one photographer, even when it was right before a performance, you danced until complete exhaustion. The madness. You believed 100 percent in your ability to move people. You continued to write love letters using your body as a brush.

You danced in forty-nine cities in Japan. You danced in ninety-eight cities in thirty other countries. Altogether, 597 performances, all after your second debut at age seventy-one! You did not calm down. You did not want to.

Though people know you as an avant-garde founder of butoh, you were also a student of two Japanese modern-dance pioneers: Baku Ishii and Takuya Eguchi. Both traveled to Germany—Ishii in 1921 and Eguchi in 1931—to study at Wigman's school and presented their pieces in Berlin. In the 1920s, Ishii performed in several other European countries and America. Your uncle, who published a bilingual book of poetry with his own pictures, spent seventeen years in America during his youth. Your aunt collected Elvis Presley albums. Your international aspirations had deep roots. You made me think, *Nobody comes from nowhere!*

After I visited China, I told you that people there would love to see you perform. You looked down and, after a long silence, said,

I can go anywhere else,
but I cannot go to China.

I realized you were there for nine years during World War II. I sensed the weight of the Japanese aggression in those who participated in the war. I appreciate that you carried your war experiences as a deep regret.

Every time you came to New York, you brought us pages of handwritten notes for each dance you performed. They are in my file cabinet. You have been here. You slept on our bed. I remember how you growled throughout the night, thinking of your dance and arguing with your son, Yoshito, who was directing you.

In 1999, in your last international appearance, you performed *Requiem for the 20th Century* at the Japan Society. You were ninety-four. You made us feel drunk, sobbing with joy. Elvis Presley was your encore. You shook your body, the theater, and us.

You loved to eat eel until the end of your life. Bedridden in your later years, you had eel smoothies for breakfast. I often imagine that eel dancing in your body.

You addressed us in your book,

Eiko & Koma, You travel with your angels.
I could not teach you anything. I thank you
and I am sorry.

Your eel dance was your “thank you” and “I am sorry” dance.

Yours,
Eiko Otake

Dear Kyra,

It has been so many years since Koma and I visited you in your house in San Francisco in 1976. When I saw the door painted bright yellow, I knew without looking at the address that it was Nijinsky's daughter's house.

I told you that *The Diary of Vaslav Nijinsky* was one of the three books I carried with me when, at age twenty, I left Japan with Koma on a ship heading for Nakhodka, Soviet Union. It was translated by dance critic Miyabi Ichikawa, who later became our friend. He introduced my teacher Kazuo Ohno to the world by bringing him to the Nancy Festival in France.

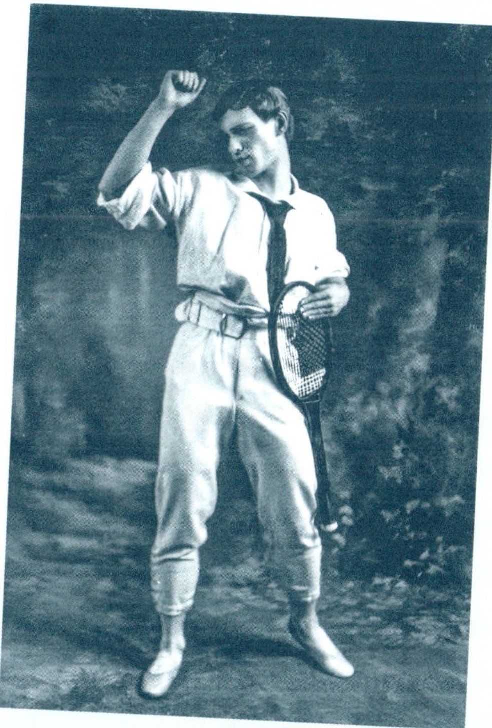

Vaslav Nijinsky, in Claude Debussy's *Les Jeux*, Ballets Russes de Diaghilev production, 1913

Kazuo Ohno and Tatsumi Hijikata, another dance artist in Japan with whom Koma and I briefly studied, spoke about Nijinsky and showed us his pictures. Your father's joyful face and slightly bent arms in *Le Spectre de la rose* were irresistible. In the first contemporary dance performance I ever saw, Hijikata used in his choreography Nijinskiy's pose from *The Afternoon of a Faun*.

Your father was a legend, a fragile beauty of insanity.

In 1973, I bought Richard Buckle's biography of Nijinsky in Amsterdam, and it was the first big book I read in its entirety in English. I understood that your father danced something more than dance. To a young dancer who was culturally and politically radicalized in a turbulent time in Japan, your father's diary illuminated how a particularly outstanding physical ability and creative drive were swallowed by war and hurtful power dynamics.

At the time, I looked but could not find any film of him dancing, which made his photographs more evocative.

Rather forcefully, you invited me to dance. I sat on your kitchen table, floated my legs and arms while balancing on my buttocks—my seaweed solo. I felt your eyes penetrating my body. Immediately after, you danced a section from *The Rite of Spring* for us. Your body, which was quite round, reminded me of many older Russian women I saw in the Soviet Union. Still, as you danced—first in your living room and then into the kitchen—your body was undoubtedly that of a dancer, moving between poses with vigorous staccato. Poetic still figures appeared between hearty stomps. Your arms were, at times, circular but turned angular. Your eyes pierced just like your father's. A dangerous glow. I saw your father coming out of his diary and living in your body. He was a giver and a victim.

You gave us a big poster of your painting of your father in *Le Spectre de la rose*. You said, "When I danced his role in this ballet, I felt how my father had felt dancing." On the poster, you wrote,

> *Dear my dance friends from far away...*
> *You danced on my kitchen table.*
>
> *My father for me was like a fairy tale. I did not need a book of fairy tales as a child because all of his ballets were my fairy tales.*
>
> *My father choreographed one way, my aunt choreographed another way, and I choreographed yet another way. But what binds us together is a family choreography, and it's the circle. That is always what my father loved, everything in circle, though he also broke out of it in his later choreography.*

In his diary, your father wrote, "The public came to be amused, and thought I danced for their amusement. My dances were frightening. They were afraid of me, thinking I wanted to kill them. I did not...I wanted to go on. But God said to me: 'Enough.' I stopped."

Dear Kyra, I cherish the memory of our meeting in the house with the yellow door.

Sincerely,
Eiko Otake

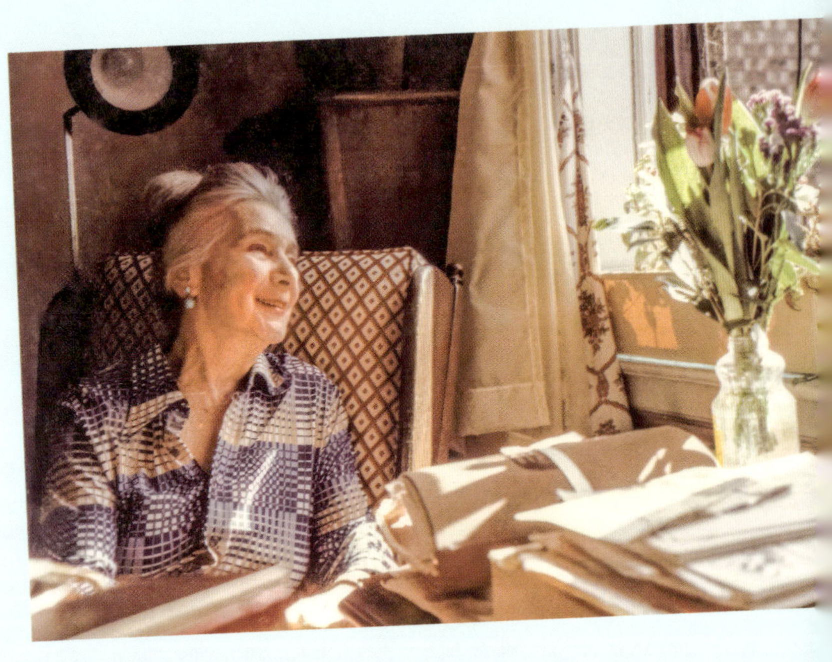

Dear Mura,

I met you at the *Dance Magazine* office soon after we came to New York in 1976. A beautiful Jewish elder, you immediately invited us to your home for tea. A New York story. You were seventy, and I was twenty-three. I was excited to become your friend. I did not know one could become a friend to someone so much older.

You were born in 1905 in Odessa, when it was a part of the Russian Empire. It is there and then that the uprising portrayed in *Battleship Potemkin* happened. Your first dance teacher, Ellen Tels, was Isadora Duncan's student. I was fascinated that you followed your teacher to Vienna in 1919 at the early age of fourteen. Your mother came to Europe with you so you could study dance, and, in 1925, you moved to Paris, where you first saw Josephine Baker, who attracted you to jazz. Such dazzling names.

I became a frequent visitor to your apartment on West 181st Street. Your home was a salon, and I met your friends: African American dancers, as well as white writers, photographers, librarians, and painters.

You told me how you felt when you entered the Savoy Ballroom soon after you came to the United States in 1930: "Dancers were dancing with such abundance and the whole floor was bouncing!" Located at 596 Lenox Avenue, between 140th and 141st Streets in Harlem, the Savoy Ballroom was where you felt an urgency to document the dancers you were dancing with. It was easy to spot you in a small section of the film you shot in the Savoy—you were the only white woman dancing in a sea of Black people, but the camera paid no special attention to you.

You told me,

> *I was a good dancer and felt completely comfortable dancing with them but Savoy dancers said, "You can surely dance but you don't dance like us." In looking back, I sacrificed my dancer and choreographer career because documenting their dancing became my work. Once I brought Herbert Matter and his camera into the Savoy, there was no turning back. I had to work with the footage. They kept dancing, creating new styles and new steps. So I had to shoot more. Producing* Spirit Moves *became my life work.*

I went to every showing of your films. To see the dancers' steps and styles, smiles and laughs. Proud exhibitions of inventions. Ease of being together but also full of vigor, sweat soaking visibly through their business suits. I was very moved. One dancer says in your film, "Spirit moves me. When the spirit leaves me, I stop dancing," thus inspiring the title of your monumental work, *The Spirit Moves*. The film's length was five hours. From these words, I thought of my teacher Kazuo Ohno, whom you also saw dance. A very different style but with the same thrust. Spirit moves body, and body moves spirit.

Seeing *The Spirit Moves* at your home and in screening events was an education. You chose the most authentic dancers to your eyes and brought them to a studio, asking them to perform earlier styles as well as new ones. Herbert Matter filmed them. They started with the cakewalk and the Charleston, before moving on to the blues, bebop, and the aerial Lindy.

You showed no hesitation in narrating the film with your European accent or adding jazz music different from what the dancers were actually dancing to. You edited directly onto 16 mm film positive—I found it all brave but scary. You confided in me, however, that the fact that you were a white person created tensions and doubts with some dancers.

Soon after we met, you came to see our performances and said,

> *Alas, you have no sense of rhythm. I can teach you!*

For some months, I took the A train after my waitress job for your jazz-dance class in your living room. You choreographed Koma and me using Patti Smith's song "Because the Night," which Patti wrote with Bruce Springsteen. After you came to the landfill on the Hudson River to see our outdoor performance in 1980, you changed your mind.

> *I think I was wrong to teach you jazz.*
> *Let me experiment on you with something else.*
> *Move your legs and feet like arms and hands.*
> *Circle your legs like fins, flutter them*
> *like wings. Roll like an injured bird.*

That was another chapter of our New York story.
I remember a carpet of yours that I rolled on.

Around that time, you gathered together young breakdancers, and I was there when you filmed them. You were a forceful and clear cheerleader with the dignity of a senior, yet a stranger to them. Your excitement with their new movement was genuine. The very young people sensed that.

Our New York story brought the biggest surprise when our son was born in 1985. Holding him, you proposed that Koma and I inherit your films. You said you worried about our son being born between us, and you pointed out we had begun creating our own films. You insisted that we inherit not only the entire film of *The Spirit Moves* but also other films you shot. I had never imagined that and protested because we came from such a different place and background. But you were firm.

This is my life work. Please note these are valuable. People will learn its value if you treat it that way.

Inheriting your films brought us a tremendous responsibility. After I made negatives of *The Spirit Moves*, I printed three copies and gave one each to the Boston Library, Paris Cinematheque, and the New York Public Library for preservation and to offer proper access to future generations. For years, the rest of your film reels were in our children's room, occupying four long, wide shelves. Now, they are all in the New York Public Library.

Two dancers from Japan with no sense of rhythm, who never danced socially, lived for decades with piles of film footage of African American people dancing in the Savoy Ballroom, other clubs, and studios. James Berry, Pepsi Bethel, Teddy Brown, Thomas King, Frankie Manning, Al Minns, Willa Mae Ricker, Sandra Gibson, Leon James, Scoby Strohman, and Esther Washington, among many others. I sincerely respect these dancers and their dancing. I feel an odd sense of personal closeness with them without ever having been among them.

When you had the first heart attack, you said, "I did not die because I had to finish editing the film." When that was done, you indeed died. Koma carried your body. The dancing body that traveled from Russia to Washington Heights. The body that danced in Europe, Harlem, and Africa. As an executor of your will, I managed your funeral. Many dancers came. You had asked me to request Mama Lou Parks to sing at your funeral. I did, and her voice rattled the funeral hall.

Thank you, Mura.

Lovingly,
Eiko

Dear Anna,

You died on May 24, 2021. I thought I had accepted that. You were one hundred years old and allowed me a delicious friendship for forty-three years. But when I got off the plane at the San Francisco International Airport recently, I had to sit down to cry. It hit me—this was the first time I had landed here and could not see you. My body remembers you.

You came to see every piece we performed in the Bay Area. You also came to see us in other cities, too. When we performed naked, which we did for many years, you teased us with a wink: "You no longer get in trouble for being naked." Your presentation of *Parades and Changes* in 1967 in New York was shut down because of its nudity, and the police issued arrest warrants for all your performers. The charge was based on New York's Blue Law, which prohibited "indecent exposure." The case went to court and was finally dismissed by a higher court.

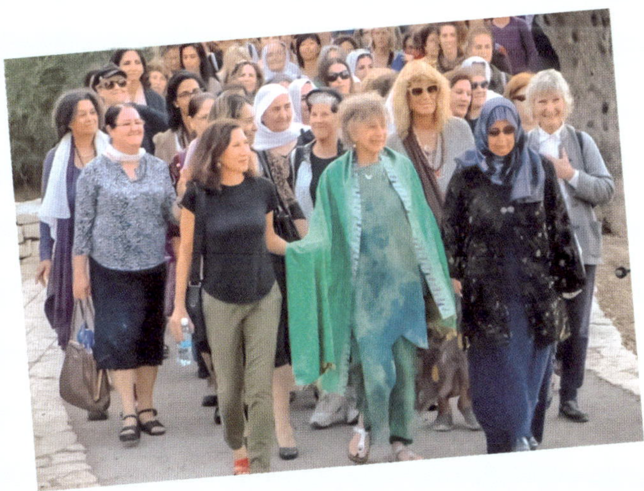

Anna Halprin leads a walking performance of Arab Israeli and Jewish Israeli women on the Haas Promenade, 2014

Thanks to you, artists, including us, could be naked without fear of arrest. I learned you created more than 150 pieces. How is that possible? I saw you scream, stomp, run, shake, and protest. I saw you nod, smile, laugh, and hug. When ridiculed as touchy-feely, you shrugged and said, “What’s wrong with that? I touch and feel!”

We first met in 1978 when you came to see our work at the San Francisco Museum of Modern Art. Right after our performance ended, you surprised me by giving us the key to your studio on Divisadero, the home of the historical San Francisco Dancers’ Workshop. You said, “You can use the studio anytime for your own rehearsals. Do you want to take my workshop? You can come as my guests.” Your first words to me revealed how you operated. You spontaneously offered a gift to us and invited these young strangers to take your class.

So Koma and I came to your workshop in your studio in Marin County. After engaging in active listening, thirty or so participants of different races and mixed abilities started to move about, each as an animal of their choice. They crawled. Some took off their clothes. Some cried. I was bewildered. Such exposure of bodies and emotion was foreign to me.

You probably knew I was uncomfortable, and that did not bother you. You had often invited critics and skeptics to dance with you. You believed in the power of dance and participation. Your student does not have to like what you do. A student can resist a teacher’s prompts, which you taught me. Though you studied with giants of modern dance, such as Martha Graham and Doris Humphrey, and even performed on Broadway, you openly criticized many choreographers and teachers.

They make others look alike and think alike. Graham said, "It takes ten years to make a dancer." But I would say it takes something like ten seconds to reveal a dancer within everyone. Anybody can be a dancer at any time when they are involved in communicating through movement.

We took another workshop in San Francisco with about a hundred people. It was the first time I saw a single woman lead so many people all day—and nobody moved in unison! You broke us into smaller groups to discuss our movement experiences. At that point, I had never been asked to speak about my movement—in neither Japan nor Europe. I realized people used simple but articulate words when they talked about their movement experiences. We also helped each other move. Your class gave me the most important principle for my teaching: movers and watchers simultaneously learn as a collective and as individuals.

Because you were so impressively vigorous, I was initially surprised to learn that you were a cancer survivor who, in everyday life, had to negotiate with your changed body. In 1972, you discovered colorectal cancer in your body. You unconsciously drew a black circle while making a self-portrait. And that led you to ask a doctor to give you a thorough examination. Your intense research into the mind-body connection articulated the distinction between a cure and healing: "A doctor could tell you you were cured of a disease, but you might not feel you were healed." When you had a recurrence in 1975, you danced to confront it, and your cancer went into remission.

Yes, Anna, our body is more ancient than any list of illnesses or medical interventions. It fears, and it wants to be consoled. And in dealing with difficulties in real life, you created new thoughts on dance and its possibilities. In the 1960s Bay Area, you were a mother, a teacher, a dancer, and an active performing artist. Your children, your students, and their mothers often performed in your work. You were keenly aware that younger generations were watching and learning from you. I love what you wrote in a 1968 pamphlet for the Marin County Dance Co-operative, where you were a teacher and organizer:

> *Where were the children at Dr. Martin Luther King's funeral? Did we adults forget that they needed to share this tragedy, to be comforted and reassured and not forgotten and ignored at a time like this? Let our children in...Let them participate together. Let them grow up and face together the tragedy and the hope of mankind.*

I find your 1970 piece *Blank Placard Dance* brilliant. After many people were repeatedly arrested in the marches, you staged a participatory protest performance on Market Street in downtown San Francisco. You divided the participants into groups of twenty-four and directed each group to walk a block apart to circumvent the law that required a permit for a gathering of more than twenty-five people! Though you continued, proudly, to get arrested, you turned a protest march into a dance with blank placards. You made an art of noncompliance and nonviolence. I wish I or others around me had your wit when our street demonstrations turned violent in Japan.

The film that documented the rehearsal of your *Ceremony of Us* (1969) shook me. How enegetically you directed the merging of a group of white people from San Francisco and a group of Black people from Studio Watts in Los Angeles. The bare skin and gaze of each person touched, slid, pushed, and pulled, creating a sensual and unnerving shimmer.

That heat and rhythm must have fueled more resolve for experimentation. You knew that one needs to be an experimentalist to seek fundamental change over the ills of the racial divide and inequality. At forty-nine, you stomped and swayed more than any other dancer, though all were far younger than you! Seeking change made you so bold and urgent. Of course, you had to value the process—rather than rehearse to create a product. These vibrations must have reached me across the ocean as the political resistance and antiwar movement swelled.

Anna, I do not want this letter to be just a remembrance or an appreciation. What I really want to say is that I am experiencing a profound strangeness regarding time. You have been my elder. But at seventy, I am moved by thinking of you when you were so much younger than I am now.

While you developed a program of healing movement work for cancer patients, AIDS arrived. In the mid-1980s, you worked with STEPS Theatre Company for People Challenging AIDS, which later became Positive Motion. The company comprised men living with AIDS and HIV when no preventive measure or cure was available to them. You said you took a long walk after each consuming session. Your teaching and your choreography were always about empathy and standing tall. The workshop led to a performance called *Carry Me Home* in 1990. As a result, certain people thought of your work as therapy, not as art—as if art should only be termed as such so narrowly. That notion could be challenged only by a dance artist who believes in the power of working and moving. YOU. You believed that change can happen when a large group of people moves with united goals. You refused to give in.

You produced large-scale works—*City Dance* (1976-77), *In and On the Mountain* (1981), *Circle the Earth* (1986-1990s), and *Planetary Dance* (1987-ongoing)—as contemporary ritual. *Planetary Dance* was produced in more than fifty places in cities worldwide, including Berlin, with four hundred participants, to commemorate the fiftieth year of the Potsdam Declaration. You told me, "Looking back on my life, I am most proud of these large-scale rituals. My most far-reaching legacy!" Anna, nobody else attempted such things, and no one else has generations of willing students to activate such ambitious ideas in so many places.

American Dance Festival produced *Circle the Earth* twice, and I loved participating in it. Hardly anyone wore a leotard. The joyful mandala of bodies in a large meadow was so different from what was usually seen on the ADF stage.

> *"I RUN FOR NO WAR!"*
> *"I RUN FOR NO DEATH PENALTY."*
> *"I RUN FOR THE LIVES OF TRANS PEOPLE."*
> *"I RUN FOR..."*

In Japan, many communities have an annual circle dance, some boasting long histories and a wide range of participants. As a child, I loved dancing in such circle dances, becoming nobody with the lure of rhythmic singing. But the Japanese dancing circle has no declaration of individual concern. No one gets to know more about the world. They dance in a circle in simple steps, uniting bodies of the same destiny.

My friend Kyoko Hayashi, who was exposed to radiation from the atomic bomb dropped on Nagasaki, described high-school students performing a circle dance in the yard of an arms factory where they had to work, helping in the war effort. Dancing among them were a few who were departing to the front. It was, for them, a ritual of departure, likely with no return. They could be killed, they could kill, or both. The dance was with no smile, only with cold sweat. Anna, your score is the opposite. Your dance is for life: it represents immersion in a community. Your public show of commitment had such rippling effects in different countries.

In January 1991, we were in the Taos Pueblo in New Mexico to see the turtle dance together. Koma and I were with our kids, visiting our collaborator Robert Mirabal. You were there with Larry. Such rituals do not start at a fixed time. You and Larry, both in your seventies, waited with us for a long time in the cold without a hint of impatience. With no camera and no notebook, you stayed to support the dancers and their prayers, which went on for hours. You told me you and Larry worked extensively with Native American people and that you had visited many Native communities to witness such rituals and to learn from their commitments. You spoke passionately: "The tribes that keep their dance alive are the ones whose languages and cultures survive. Dance is a major force. Not only does a dancer make a dance, but a dance also makes a dancer. Dancers grow with a commitment as both individuals and as community members."

In 2000, upon receiving a Kennedy Center commission, Koma proposed, "How about collaborating with Anna?" I knew Larry was not well and that would be an obstacle. I was, therefore, surprised when you said yes at my first asking. We agreed that all rehearsals would be held in your studio over several visits. The following year, 9/11 made the situation tense. Our premiere was the same week anthrax was found in the Capitol. You were eighty-one, Koma was fifty-three, and I was forty-nine. We performed

Be With at the Kennedy Center in Washington, DC; Yerba Buena Center for the Arts in San Francisco; and the Joyce Theater in New York. The last turned out to be your first public performance in New York since the warrant for your arrest was issued in 1967.

Working in your studio and making a piece together was a very different experience from taking your classes. I felt your body still held so much of American modern dance, its culture and technique; I had so little of that in my body. You rebelled against some aspects, and you embraced some. But your body remembered, and they surfaced when we were working together. It was as if working with us made you act more like the American you were. You put two arms together and straight up, looking at your hands and then to the sky like Isadora! I moved my arms hesitantly and separately. I felt shy to straighten them or to look at my hands or the sky.

I grew up in postwar Japan and protested the Vietnam War, so I had a distaste for loud and cheerful Americanness. My grandmothers and two aunts professionally danced Japanese traditional dance, in which straight and symmetrical shapes are rare. I showed you my grandfather's paintings and how bodies, movements, and poses were depicted with nuance. In return, you said how inspired you were looking at your grandfather in the synagogue:

> *As my grandfather prayed, he chanted in Hebrew and swayed back and forth. As his prayers intensified, he would clap his hands, fling them into the air, and jump about. Although I didn't understand what he was saying, I felt his voice and movements within my body. I felt his passion and heart, and I intuitively understood that he was dancing.*
>
> *Jews are a dancing people.*

You were delighted when I shared my egg exercise: On the floor, we traveled together beyond our cultural and historical memories, lying, moving, and imagining before we were born—as an egg and sperm forming cellularly into different body parts that could function as a stomach, cheek, or armpit.

I saw your solo *From 5 to 110* in your seventy-fifth-birthday performance in 1995.

> *When I was forty, I danced for social justice and peace...*
> *When I became half of a hundred, I became very ill.*
> *I thought I would die...*
> *When I am one hundred, I will dance the essence of things.*

At eighty-nine, you taught a huge, sold-out class sponsored by Movement Research at Judson Church. All day, you never once sat down. I remember you spoke firmly: "People say I am a pioneer of postmodern dance. I do not know what the hell they are talking about—I just dance! There are two ways to look at movement: one is when a mind informs a body. But there are ways a body can inform a mind."

In 2014, at age ninety-four, you traveled to Israel to lead a ritual—an all-female silent peace walk on the Haas Promenade, which Larry codesigned with Shlomo Aronson. True to your vision, women from Israel, Palestine, Russia, and Ukraine walked tightly together. Upon hearing your vivid report, I felt shame that I had tried to discourage you from taking such a long trip at that age. You never calculated or saved your energy when you wanted to do something.

Even in difficult circumstances, you never allowed yourself or others to lose hope.

On November 10, 2016, soon after the presidential election Donald Trump won, I received an email that you sent to people all over the world:

> *THE "MOURNING" AFTER THE ELECTION SCORE*
> *· ENTER, SAY HELLO*
> *· FIND A SPOT, CRASH*
> *· PICK YOURSELF UP, BRUSH YOURSELF OFF*
> *· PRAY*
> *· MOVE FORWARD*
>
> *Peace,*
> *Anna*

Anna, you demonstrated what it is to mentor many people in times of difficulty.

In 2019, I had a great two-day visit with you. You were ninety-nine years old and still teaching.

I said goodbye to you on October 17, 2019. My last visit.

How many hundreds or perhaps thousands studied with you? People from different generations and different countries with different trajectories. Many of them now work independently and teach. They raise children and build communities. Your voice remains loud and clear. I too want to shout. I too want to shout LOUD. Justice but no revenge! No killing.

THANK YOU, ANNA!

Yours truly,
Eiko

March 13, 2024

When did you first witness dance? Where was it? Who or what was dancing? Who or what were they dancing with? How long were you there? Was there music? Can you still hear the music? Was it on purpose? Was it a performance? Or were you a voyeur? What moved them? Did you move? Did you want to move? What stopped the movement? How far is this dance from you now? Do you need it now? Do you remember a phrase, a combination, an eight count?

1-2.

On balls of feet. Right foot steps forward and crosses body at a slight diagonal. Both hands are flexed with left elbow bent and hand up and right elbow straight with hand down at side.

3-4.

Switch. Left foot steps forward and crosses body at a slight diagonal. Right elbow is bent with hand up and left elbow is straight with hand down at side.

5-6.
Repeat 1-2.

7-8.
Repeat 3-4.

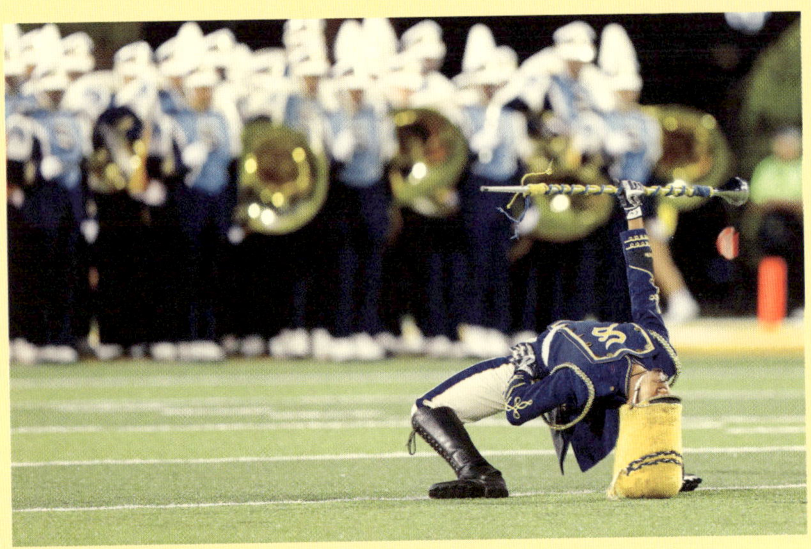

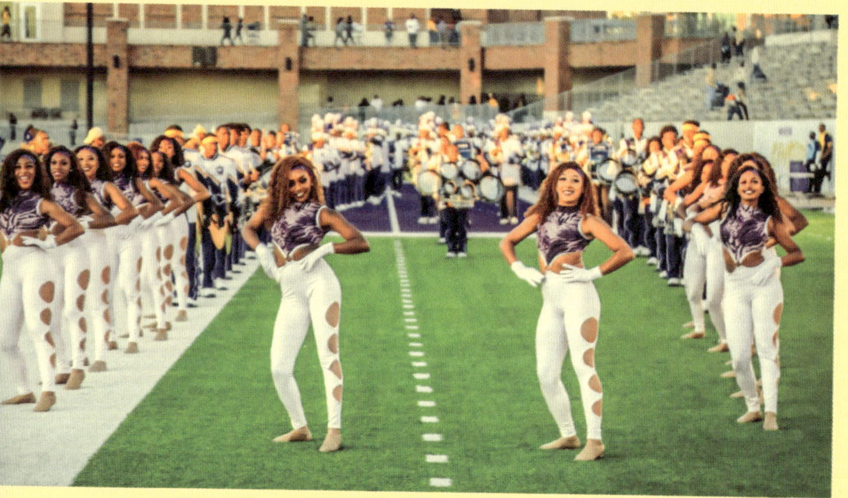

Southern University's marching band, Human Jukebox, Southern Miss Golden Eagles vs. Southern University Jaguars, M. M. Roberts Stadium, September 9, 2017. Photo: © Chuck Cook–USA TODAY Sports

Prairie View A&M University's Black Foxes, Prairie View A&M University vs. Jackson State University, Independence Stadium, Shreveport, Louisiana, October 26, 2013. Photo: Marching Storm Media

The coveted opening ceremony of any Black Southern football game is the marching in of drum majors, majorette dancers, and the band. The game is played on the field, but the attention is here. The drum majors range in formality. They might don T-shirts and track pants or the full marching-band regalia, complete with capes, gloves, spats, boots, and shakos, leading the line with their batons in hand. When the drum majors step onto the field, the stadium comes alive. Their movement is rooted in an open, swinging pelvis, a low center of gravity, and high knees.

Drum majors move in dialogue with the main event: the majorette dancers. These predominantly Black femme teams perform alongside the marching band at weekly football and basketball games, homecomings, and battle-of-the-bands competitions. They emerge in precise lines, led by the captain. They are shrouded in metallics. Spandex camisoles, jazz pants, booty shorts, tight leotards with billowing skirts, and detached forearm sleeves and gloves, complemented by nude tights tucked into jazz or character shoes. Hair is a part of the uniform, often silk-pressed and bumped into bouncy, layered, shoulder-length curls. It can be bought or come straight out of the head. It just needs to swing. Glossed lips part for wide smiles that won't be dropped until the evening is done.

The majorettes enter with a strut. Each team's is unique. They may rise onto the balls of their feet or keep them planted on the ground. They may sway their hips with speed or keep their pelvis pointed forward. They may raise their arms above their heads or swing them forward and back parallel to the hips. The details of the strut belong to the captain and dancers. This entrance announces the performance and sets the tone of what's to come.

The marching band follows the majorettes. The musicians come immaculately dressed: tailored jackets and pants in their school colors, adorned with their school crest, shakos with plumes (a feather), and marching shoes. They arrive in strict lines and cut shapes through the space, carving sharp edges along their path. The drumline

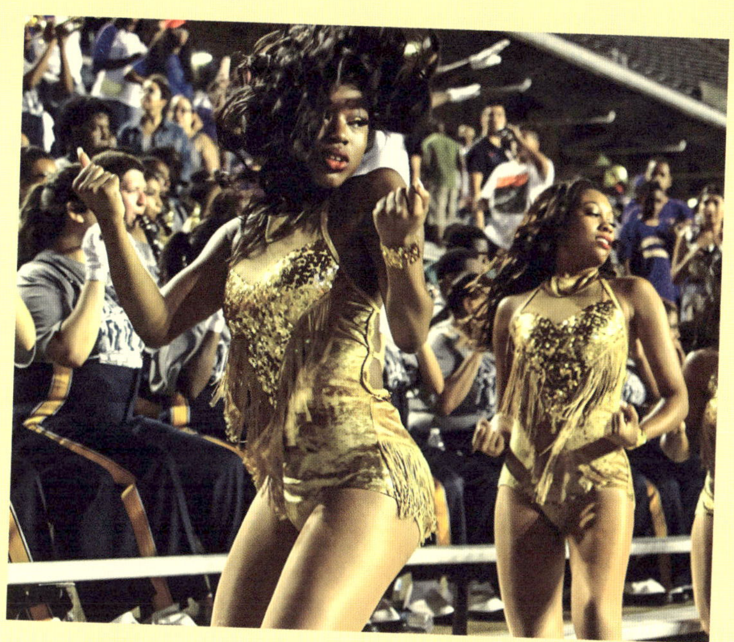

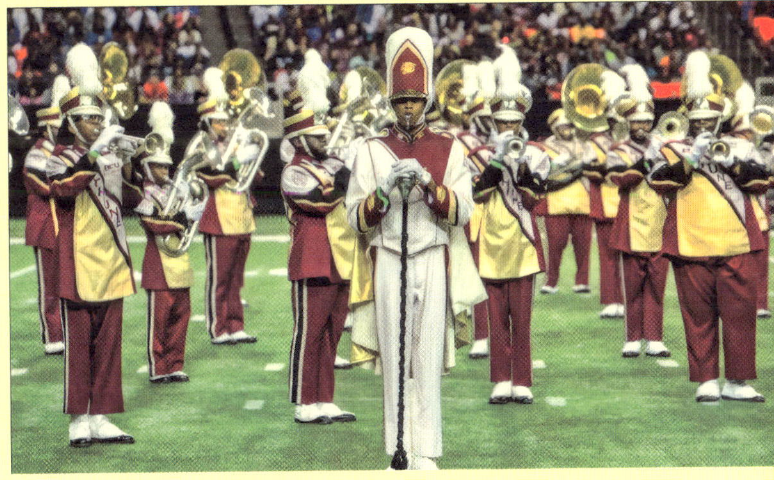

Prairie View A&M University's Black Foxes, Prairie View A&M University vs. Rice University Owls, Rice Stadium, Houston, August 25, 2018. Photo: 2C2K Photography

Bethune-Cookman University's Marching Wildcats, Honda Battle of the Bands, Georgia Dome, Atlanta, January 30, 2016. Photo: Jewel Wicker, courtesy of Honda comes first, followed by the brass and wood instruments. The band transforms rap, hip-hop, and R & B songs with distinctive melodies into percussive, horn-heavy soundscapes. They move with the sound, instruments shifting with their choreography. Witnesses rock along to the music at the encouragement of the drum majors and majorettes, married to the beat. The eight count is coveted. Attention is held.

The entire line follows the track's path, and they make their way into the stands.

> Upon reaching the risers,
> stand with left foot beveled.
> Hands on hips.
> Elbows should form sharp edges.

In the context of the Deep South and Black schools, majorettes are simply called "dance team." This is dance outside of a purely social context. It distills and explodes a variety of forms—jazz, hip-hop, contemporary, and musical theater—by taking a wholly Black approach. Combinations are led by the captain, who performs an eight-count solo, prompting the rest of the team to do so in a canon. "Watch me," the captain says, signaling the act with two fingers pointed at their own eyes. The team moves in step with the marching band. They must remain in character, smile and glowing gaze unchanged, even when sitting in the stands between combinations.

Majorettes build a formal ecosystem that is hypnotic to watch. This is most clearly seen in the hierarchy of the captain position. This coveted role highlights a dancer with exceptional musicality, a sense of timing, stamina, and performative presence. The captain grounds the group. They lead the line during the opening strut. Once in the stands, they are perched in their own row with the rest of the team elevated behind them. They execute each combination first, establishing the tempo and emotional tone each section will take. Their movements must be fluid, pouring forth effortlessly but majestically, imploring the other dancers to do the same. The captain is loyal to the band, beginning a set of combinations at the start of a song and finishing shortly after the end, falling into the potent aftermath of the music. The rigor of the entire system continues in the formations from the strut to the stands, the allegiance to the count, the detail of the movement, and the uniformity of both hair and costume. This is tradition. This is ritual.

The majorettes are the energetic fuel behind these football games. When gathering around this intense display of masculine energy, the source of power in Black community is revealed: we are most drawn to and held together by Black femmes. Although relegated to the stands, they enchant the entire stadium, filled with tens of thousands of people. They manifest magic through specificity. There are clear objectives, physically and emotionally, behind each eight count. And the dancers always hit.

As in most Black formal and social dance practices, the core of majorette movement is undulation. That controlled roll slips through the dancers. It moves through the arch of the foot, slithers up the thighs, hugs the hips, scoops out the pelvis, and envelops the back. It travels from the captain through the entire line. With each sway

1. Hands, flexed, emerge first. Pump right arm forward, lift out of hip.

2. Pull right arm back, pump left arm forward, sink into hip.

3. Pump right arm up, pull left arm in, lift out of hip.

4. Pull right arm back, pump left arm up, sink into hip.

5. Left arm remains up. Pump right arm forward, sink into hip.

6. Draw a semicircle with the right arm, sinking into hip when it reaches the right side of the body.

7. Repeat step 5.

8. Repeat 6.

and throw, they sink deeper into the deeply set edges of the combination. Each limb and look knows where to land. The dancers bounce. They are open yet controlled. They are the definition of smooth.

Alongside undulation is stillness. They wait without anticipation. The period between combinations is elevated by severe poses: upright, chest forward, chin up, and hands organized royally. That stillness holds the entire stadium's attention as the fans savor what they have just witnessed. The journey repeats: from undulation to stillness, undulation to stillness.

Three performances give clear examples of this movement quality and the conditions that surround it.

The first shows Alabama State University's Sensational Stingettes at a battle of the bands competition. The majorettes and marching band take center stage. Here, the dancers come to attention in an upright pose with one hand on the hip and the other extended sharply forward. A few seconds into

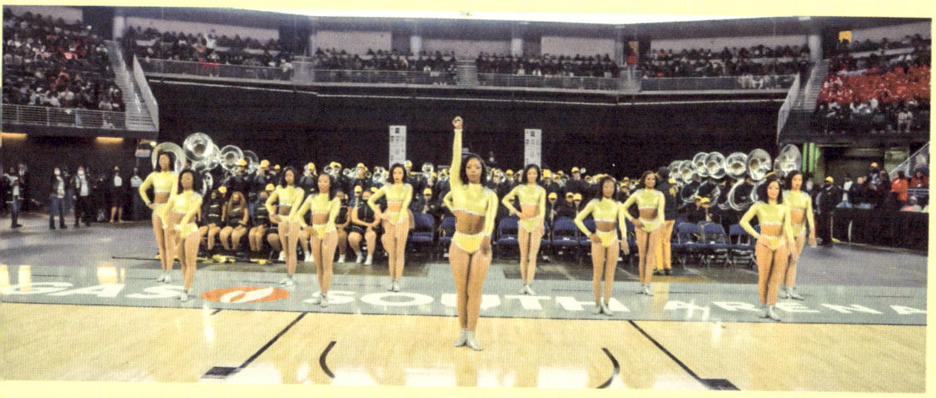

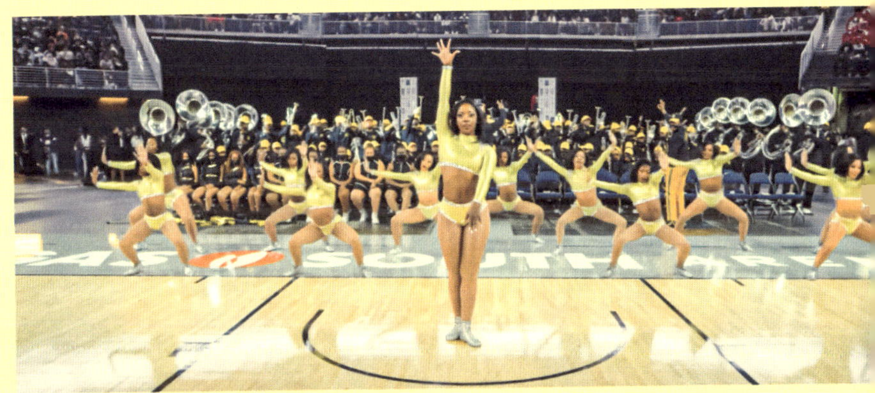

Alabama State University's Sensational Stingettes, HBCU Culture Battle of the Bands, Bojangles Coliseum, Charlotte, North Carolina, November 6, 2022

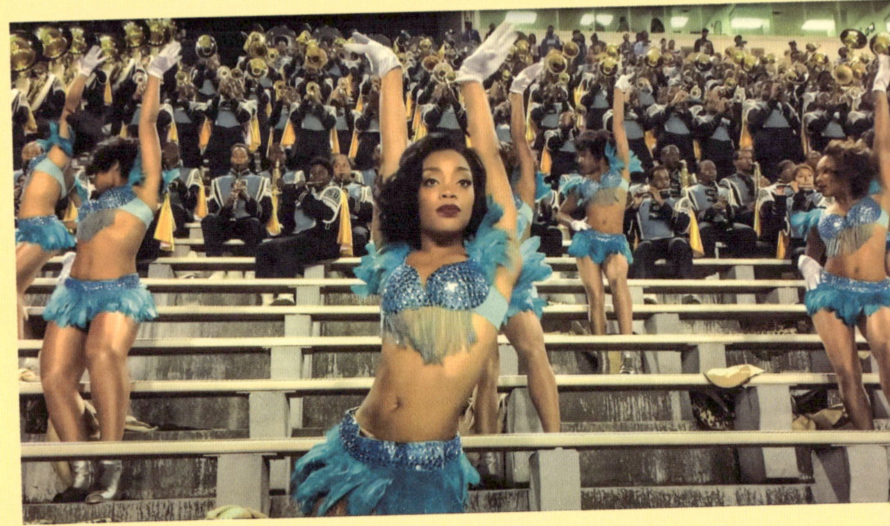

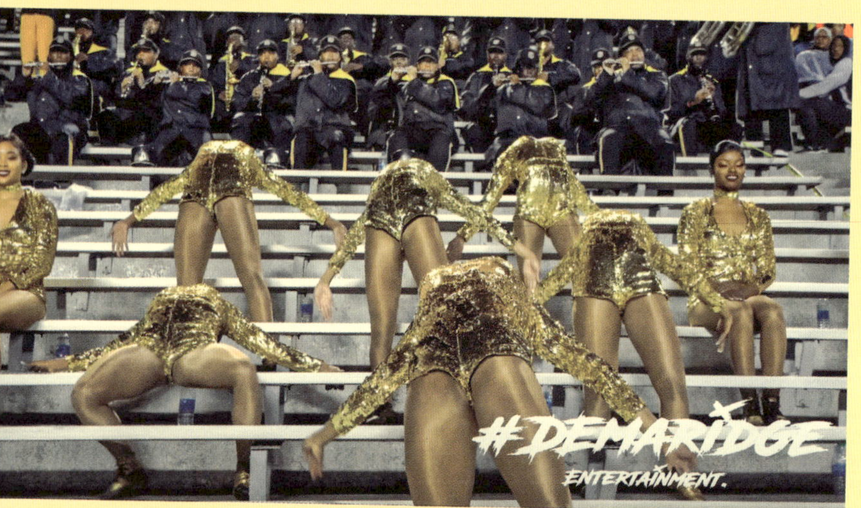

Southern University's marching band, Human Jukebox, and Dancing Dolls, Southern University vs. Texas Southern University, A. W. Mumford Stadium, Baton Rouge, Louisiana, November 8, 2014. Still from Trin.T Productions YouTube channel

Alabama State University's Marching Hornets and Sensational Stingettes at the Magic City Classic, Birmingham, Alabama, October 26, 2019. Still from Demaridge YouTube channel the performance, the dancers rip out of this position and into a grounded, low thrust. The drum majors often take on this swinging pelvis, a riotous action that appears to charge up the performers before they push that energy outward. This moment is beautifully aggressive and seemingly masculine. The dancers break the fluid shifts of their choreography to push against the expectations of how a pack of politely postured femmes should dance.

Next are the Southern University Dancing Dolls and their performance to "Can You Stand the Rain" by New Edition. One of the most prolific majorette teams among the HBCUs (Historically Black Colleges and Universities), the Dancing Dolls embody a spirit of controlled seduction. Their movement oscillates between rich softness and ferocity, an oscillation further pronounced by their outfits: they are adorned in vibrant blue enlivened by feathers, sequins, silk gloves, and tassels. With sartorial choices reminiscent of Josephine Baker, the Dancing Dolls put forth a similar command and employment of femininity. Their captain slips into the smoothness of the song. She is both activating and activated by the music. The song choice is a classic. And it allows for one of the most exciting moments in these performances: recognizing the music. The majorettes help the audience enter the melody. You want to know what song it is as quickly as those around you. You want to enter the collective excitement of enjoying it in a new form. You are gifted new music out of the old. Will it move you too?

Finally, the Sensational Stingettes at Arizona State University, who always dazzle in gold, are this time costumed in sequined rompers with their hair pulled back to let the outfits shine. While this performance exemplifies a skill like that of the Dancing Dolls, I want to highlight a mistake. Early on in a collective eight count, six dancers throw their heads back and their arms to the sides. One of the dancers loses her balance and slips back onto the bleachers. But her recovery is seamless. Majorettes have to stay on count. There are no individual decisions to the beat. The beauty of the performance is the synchronization, the exactitude. This dancer stays true to that requirement. She picks herself back up without a fuss and

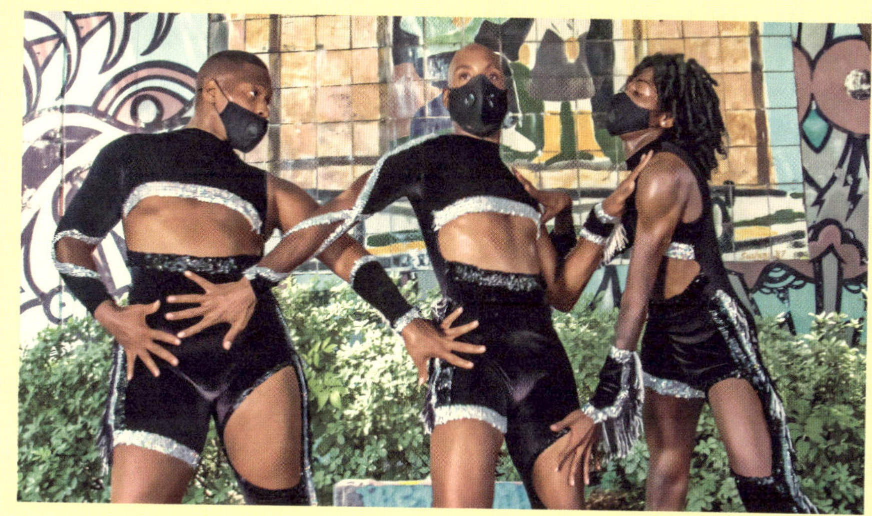

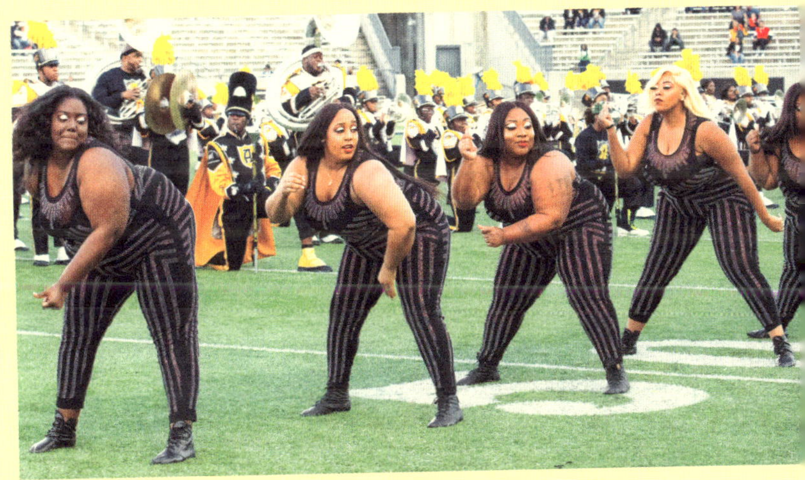

Darrius Stephens, Leland Thorpe, and Ter'Schard Harris of Dance Champz of Atlanta pose in front of Steve Seaberg's mosaic *The Fiddler*, Atlanta, August 16, 2020. Still from *J-Setting: From Southern HBCUs to the Clubs of Atlanta* by Frederick Taylor (director) and Yusef Ferguson (cinematographer)

Alabama State University's alumni Honey Beez, performing during halftime at Alabama State University vs. Prairie View A&M University, Alabama State Stadium, Montgomery, November 28, 2019. © Kirsten Fiscus–USA TODAY NETWORK does not miss any of the following counts. You can't help but be proud of her. This moment of vulnerability cuts through the challenge of perfection. She is exceedingly intimidating, then immensely human.

In recent decades, majorette practice has expanded into increasingly liberatory forms. J-setting, which originated with the Prancing J-Settes at Jackson State University in Mississippi during the 1970s, has been embraced by the queer Black community in response to the often all-female cisgender exclusivity of majorette teams. Then there is Alabama State University's Honey Beez dance team, created by band director James Oliver in 2004 as a fat-positive alternative to the Sensational Stingettes. As with any form, there is so much the practice has yet to learn, so many parts of tradition it must be willing to break.

Black Southern majorette dancers have codified a particular power: Black femme sensuality organized into eight counts. Within this sensuality is a seductive movement quality and an outward persona that commands attention,

2. Sit into right hip with left knee popped. Both hands are resting on the back of the head, elbows bent.

1. Trace the floor and draw right leg back while swinging right arm out alongside it.

3. Pop left hip up.

4. Sit back into right hip.

5. Drop torso down over legs and slap thighs.

6. Roll up, butt sticking out, elbows bent with hands resting above butt.

7. Step back and pop right knee out.

8. Step back and pop left knee out.

leaving you entranced. This sensuality also offers the opportunity for pleasure in oneself. The dancers perform without directing their gaze or attention to any individual. Instead, the dancers are providing audiences with the opportunity to tune in and imagine themselves as the direct recipients of these dances. Their gaze is somehow both external and internal. Dropping, rolling, and coiling, they wrap themselves up in their own sensual journey.

These femmes are active decision-makers, cultural icons, rigorous creatives, and so much more. They dramatically perform femmeness, reclaiming an identity that is often exploited or degraded in environments of subjugation. This is an opportunity to imagine gender expression as a bonding agent for a community rather than an individual trait. Majorettes hold femmeness up to the light and deliberately choose how they will employ it through each count. This is Black femmes in their autonomy. This is Black femmes in their power. This is Black femmes in their radical presence. When the captain moves, the world stops. We want to see more of what they have for us.

1. Standing with legs hip-width apart, open arms out to the sides of the body.

2. Swivel right arm over head and bring both hands to the right hip.

3-4. Placing one hand on top of the other, swing both arms over and around head and rest them on left hip. Head is looking over left shoulder.

5. Turn head to look over right shoulder.

6. Switch hands from left hip to right hip. Sit into right hip.

7. Throw both arms up over head, hands still connected. Rock pelvis forward.

8. Step legs out hip-width apart, with knees bent. Hands slap down to knees. Throw pelvis/butt backward.

Black femmes, queer and trans folks, women, and birthing people continue to lose opportunities for autonomy. Amid darkening civil landscapes, dance for dance's sake is a necessary somatic release. But I am reaching a step further, wanting to immerse myself in the profound cultural context of Blackness and the Deep South. I do not value our formal governing bodies. I value the rules of majorette practice. Majorette dance is a system for being. It's clarity. It's history. It's affirmation.

I am immersed in a contemporary dance field that credits "groove" to Ohad Naharin, a white Israeli choreographer art-washing the belligerent occupation of Palestine. Anne Teresa De Keersmaeker's work with her purposefully thin, predominately white, all-female company, Rosas, is praised as pioneering complex counts, repetition, and layering. And Trisha Brown, arguably the most significant inspiration behind the continued reliance on a lethargic postmodern white-girl aesthetic, is considered innovative for the deliberate use of gesturing and posturing in public space. Contemporary dance thought it was witnessing individual breakthroughs. Meanwhile, the majorette community was hitting all these marks in HBCU football stadiums.

1. Pop left leg out at a diagonal. One arm is raised higher than the other, elbows bent, palms facing out. Lift out of the right hip. Arms switch heights. Sit into the right hip. /// 2. Repeat 1. /// 3. Step forward on right foot, swinging arms and torso down over knees. /// 4. Step back into position from count 1. /// 5-6. Swing left leg back and pop right knee out. Throw hands out to the side, palms facing down. /// 7-8. Drop arms and take two steps to return to facing forward.

I am not an expert at this. But I write about majorettes for the same reason I compulsively watch majorette videos—to try to get it back. Dance first left an impression on me when I witnessed majorettes at my hometown football games. They were the only dancers I knew, and majorette dance is the first form I learned. These Black femmes were the captains of all dance. In them, I could see my own Black femme body throwing, snapping, rolling, stretching, and posing with such fire. Over the years, I tasted and upheld new forms and styles of dance that removed majorettes from the forefront of my knowledge. I didn't return to that training. I didn't pour into it, roll through it, mark out its edges past the age of fourteen. I didn't codify it in my body. Instead of continuing my majorette training, led by my seventh-grade math teacher, Ms. Miller, I learned Ohad, Anne, and Trisha. I took post-modern, contemporary, and ballet classes. I performed and auditioned in these styles. And to do so, I often had to abandon my body—what it once knew and where it was shaped. It never fit. And I forgot where it did.

I am attempting to hold in one body how I dance now and how I danced then. How did I want to dance then, and how do I want to dance now? We can see a dance, know a dance, love a dance, learn a dance, but what makes it our dance? How do I pull majorettes out of teenage nostalgia and into my present-day intuitive mode of moving? My memory is spotty. Perhaps this digest isn't to be trusted.

My dances are now attempts at regaining what I thought I saw, what I thought I was, and asserting how I want to be. So, too, is this text.

When did you first witness dance? Have you returned to that dance? Have you desired to? Can you name that desire? Can you legitimize it? Have you danced this desire back into your body? Dance is an opportunity to physicalize our memories. We can root our dancing when we name that memory and desire. We can find future dances by emulating past ones. We can acknowledge the break. We might not regain the specificity of that introduction, but we can make the process of stitching these selves an idiosyncratic practice.

So I enter the stands for a Friday-night football game in Tucker, Georgia, on the suburban outskirts of Atlanta. I pack into the benches alongside Black families outfitted in their finest school spirit. I hear the hum of excitement for what is to come. I lean forward. Peer down. The rubber track is filling with a group of ornately dressed performers. Arranged at the front are two parallel lines of Black femmes, fronted by a single dancer breaking center.

1-2.

On balls of feet. Right foot steps forward and crosses body at a slight diagonal. Both hands are flexed with left elbow bent and hand up and right elbow straight with hand down at side.

3-4.

Switch. Left foot steps forward and crosses body at a slight diagonal. Right elbow is bent with hand up and left elbow is straight with hand down at side.

5-6.
Repeat
1-2.

7-8.
Repeat
3-4.

Upon reaching the risers, stand with left foot beveled. Hands on hips. Elbows form sharp edges.

The captain raises her hand. I hop a few bleachers down and slide closer to the formation of glittering gold.

"Watch me."

People ask me how I started dancing and when. When did dancing begin? It is folly to attempt to articulate the beginning of anything, but it is righteous for any dancer to claim a history.

+++

A history of dancing is a history of people in search of freedom.

A history of dancing is flooded with attempts to ground and home under conditions of displacement, migration, and diaspora. Fleeing very different forms of constraint, Josephine Baker, Isadora Duncan, and Vaslav Nijinsky all landed in Paris in the early twentieth century. Though all three artists were caught in orientalist traps (exotification and appropriation of other cultures), projecting mythical fantasias that exist only in the perverted colonial imagination, they each, in their own ways, subverted norms of gender, sexuality, and class in their embodiment of a new aesthetics in which their bodies could be freer. Baker's dancing celebrated jazz, Africanist aesthetics, Black social dance, queerness, Black autonomy in Paris, empowered female sexuality, and the Black diva. Duncan embodied first-wave feminism with bare legs, no corset, no bra, and political speeches against marriage. And Nijinsky choreographed homoeroticism and folkloric fantasias for the Ballet Russes.

My teacher Lucas Hoving was on tour with the German choreographer Kurt Joos performing the legendary antiwar dance *The Green Table* when World War II broke out, trapping Lucas outside Europe. After joining the Dutch Armed Forces in exile, he eventually settled in New York, where he became a key member of José Limón's company.

Mary Wigman fled the war from Germany to "neutral" Switzerland, where she trained with Rudolf von Laban at

Monte Verità and was exposed to Dada artists and the Cabaret Voltaire in Zurich. From these travels, she brought us a modern dance of elbows, angles, vulvas, floorwork, and the haunting potential of vintage clothing.

Charya Burt and her generation of master teachers of Cambodian classical dance taught in fear and secrecy under the genocidal regime of the Khmer Rouge or fled to the United States, risking everything to save and protect their dance lineage and technique, starting schools and companies in multiple cities in California. Burt's is a dance of remembering/mourning, a dancing-in-exile that is simultaneously a dance of creating home and community in diaspora.

Wars on Indigenous culture forced Native American and First Nations artists to migrate from tribal areas and communities to cities. Displaced by residential schooling and tribal-termination policies, urban Indians organized the 1969 occupation of Alcatraz, which inspired current generations of Native art, dance, and performance.

Gays and queers like me have sought refuge from the wars in family, home, church, school, and nation, migrating to cities in which queer cultures have blossomed despite persecution. I come from a long line of small-town queers who fled to San Francisco to dance.

A history of dance is a history of social dancing.

In 1978, Marie Hélène Benais and I, both eighteen, won the Canadian National Jitterbug competition. There were few competitors because almost no one bothered traveling to Sudbury, my smallish hometown in Northern Ontario, located on the traditional lands of the Atikameksheng Anishnawbek First Nation. Marie and

I had been dancing partners for two or three years, focused primarily on heteronormative, gendered revival dances from the fifties (jive, jitterbug); we had an acrobatic style with a lot of lifts, for which I spun Marie off the ground or around my body. We rehearsed in our school hallway, at the foot of the stairs, where our clique of freaks—smart girls, closeted queers, theater kids, fat kids—ate lunch to avoid the conformity and cruelty of the cafeteria. A rejuvenating and life-affirming spirit lives inside shared stepping, kicking, clapping, and moving.

Years later, after I moved to the United States, I learned about the Lindy hop and the Black roots of the fifties rock 'n' roll dances we had enjoyed. Sometime around the 1977 release of *Saturday Night Fever*, Marie and I pivoted to competitive disco dancing. The music, fashion, and dance innovations of disco were also appropriated from or deeply influenced by the generative yet often problematic confluence of Black social dance and gay and queer lineages and legacies.

A history of dance is a history of AIDS.

Decades after my competitive disco dancing and moving to San Francisco in 1982, I began to teach the hustle in my contemporary-dance classes. I play the Trammps's "Disco Inferno" at high volume and start the four-directional line dance. When everyone has the basics down, I turn the music off and report that "somewhere between one quarter and one-third of the people I danced with in San Francisco clubs in the early to mid-1980s were dead of AIDS by 1996. For me, disco dancing, especially the hustle, is akin to a ghost dance, an ancestor dance." There is usually a somber silence, a sharp contrast to the party mood generated by the music and communal dancing.

My history of dancing is very entangled with a history of AIDS. By that, I mean with a history of illness, dying, death, fears of male-male intimacy, governmental betrayal, die-ins, candlelight vigils, and a cultural queeruption—memories of which are activated in my body when I hear disco music, when I teach students the hustle, or when I am asked about dance history.

These are just a few of the many dancers whose AIDS-related deaths broke my heart: Gryphon Blackswan, whose drag performances demonstrated an intimacy I aspired to, using a fur stole to cover his Hickman port in a moving drag lip-synch at a Billie Gathering no/talent show; Joah Lowe, my first dance teacher in San Francisco; Craig Marquette: "It was Craig's death that galvanized my embrace of agitprop," choreographer Rick Darnell of the High Risk Group once texted me; Ed Mock: the first and most liberated solo improviser I ever witnessed; Peter Kadyk, who replaced me and wore my clothes in Contraband; Aaron Osborne, the cofounder of Dancers' Group and Footwork Studio, where I took classes with Lucas Hoving in the eighties and where years later we slept on a hard studio floor during a three-day occupation to protest the nonprofits' eviction during the first dot-com boom; Tracy Rhoades, a choreographer I knew was going to be great and after whose memorial we had an awkward orgy; James Tyler, who co-created Mariposa Studio, where I would spend a decade dancing with Sara Shelton Mann and Contraband, and the only gay founding member of Mangrove, an early all-men's contact-improvisation collective; Reza Abdoh; Alvin Ailey; Jerome Caja; Oskrr Earthsong-Feino; Philip-Dimitri Galas; Hibiscus; Cruz Luna; Rudolf Nureyev; Diet Popstitute; Purusha; John Shaw; Sylvester; Gene Williams; David Wojnarowicz; Arnie Zane... I don't want to stop writing these names.

A history of dance is a history of making families.

The dance that changed everything for me was *EVOL*, a 1985 choreography by Sara Shelton Mann created with a new company, Contraband. Mann's work is collaborative, and in the 1980s, Contraband would spend up to a year developing a new performance. It was primarily unpaid labor: we all worked freelance jobs to enable us to rehearse three days a week in the studio for two to three hours. When it was time to present the piece, we did all the work ourselves—production, promotion, PR, ticketing, street posters, and cleanup. Bathed in fire and wind, *EVOL* (*LOVE* spelled backward) was an initiatory rite for Contraband, shifting how we saw ourselves and presented ourselves to the world. In our raggedy, secondhand, black-and-white clothes and punked hair, we danced ferociously, recited absurd poetry, and sang as a barbershop trio. I wore a skirt, and every night Sara used a hatchet to smash a wooden table, a symbol of family civility, until it collapsed. The project and the artists involved were well received by those at the cultural margins. We had instant community.

A history of dance is a history of relating and collaboration.

Making a dance is uniquely intimate. The erotics and politics of collaboration are foregrounded in the studio, where breath and sweat, proximity and touch, scent and sensation, and culture and identity are closely entangled. Our dances reveal how we make and remake personal boundaries to avoid harm, protect our shame, and defend our rights.

In collaboration, we struggle for power, voice, and influence. Some of that friction is generative. We arrive at decisions together and yield to the decisions that the situation necessitates. When collaborating with folks who do not share dancing experiences—musicians, presenters, designers, tech crew—dancers negotiating creative and logistical issues are frequently misunderstood. Sentences collapse under the weight of inarticulable modes of perception and the impossibility of translation from movement to language. Dancing practices generate alternative ways to communicate and listen: focusing attention, expanding awareness, and activating senses. The studio is a laboratory for developing social relations. Multidisciplinary choreographer Kevin O'Connor has talked about collaboration as a willingness to be changed by others. This is both the promise and the danger of collaboration. The anarchist Gustav Landauer (1870–1919) once said, "The State is a condition, a certain relationship between human beings, a mode of behavior; we destroy it by contracting other relationships, by behaving differently toward one another." I watch students struggle with the word *destroy*, replacing it with *transform*, while defending the need for some structures of (political) behavior to be dismantled. Together, we expand Landauer to account for our relations with nonhumans and to activate our ecological and spiritual imaginations. Among the behaviors and relationships that need to be renegotiated, human-plant relations might be regarded as a shared breath with those of rivers, mountains, objects, and buildings.

How can improvised dancing, framed as a political practice, help unwind supremacist or neoliberal embodiments that make collaboration and equity difficult or impossible? Contact-improvisation innovator Steve Paxton has suggested that the improvising duet might be the smallest possible research unit for experiments in democracy. How might we make consensual decisions, prioritizing yielding and shared momentum rather than initiation or leadership? Contact improvisation is typically practiced as a duet between two dancers in physical contact. Sensing and yielding to each other through touch and shared weight, the dancers might roll on the floor like puppies, catch one another in dramatic lifts, or pause to explore the micro-movements of stillness. CI dancing happens in both professional and hobbyist contexts, most frequently at weekly jams and annual festivals. In 1979, in contact improvisation classes in Montréal, I learned the physical techniques and creative practices that shaped my physical body, inspired my relational body, and activated my political attention. Contact classes experimented with somatic practices that prioritize body sensations over body shapes, guiding me into tracking these sensations while touching, playing with, and rolling over a dance partner. Erotic activity was resonant, only a razor's edge away. And although I found my sexuality through contact improvisation, I was closeted in these predominantly hetero jam spaces for my first few years. I wrestled with the tension between CI's embodiment of heteronormative whiteness and its more radical potential, succinctly articulated by daniel mang in 2021: "From the beginning, I saw contact as an implicit criticism of how bodies are lived and experienced, touch used, longing organized, in patriarchal, racist…class societies, and as containing a radical utopian potential for alternative ways of embodiment."

Alongside philosophies of anarchism, participatory democracy, and feminism, collaborative dance improvisation can question how power structures enable domination and violence. In her Parable series, Octavia Butler writes, "All that you touch, you change. All that you change, changes you." My dance family tree of lovers and collaborators, companies and collectives, friendships, and queered kinships that have changed my work, identity, and perceptions include 848 Community Space, Blank Map, Cahin-Caha/cirque bâtard, CI jams, Circo Zero, Contraband, CORE, Millions of Dots/Group Rhythm Therapy, St. Urbain Lunchbox, Tell, TRY, Turbulence, and countless duet partners.

A history of dance is a history of urban real estate.

The speculative space. The artist's loft. The collective warehouse. The former garage. The shuttered can factory, the sweatshop, the public school. Improvisation in the city. Exploiting the abandoned cracks within forms of class warfare that have created failed neighborhoods, food deserts, toxic concentration, and racial segregation.

Dancers gather in these spaces, prioritizing a life of dance over family, housing security, economic stability, and privacy. We love a good floor. A history of dance is a history of cold studios, inadequate studios, shared studios, too-small studios, impossible-to-clean-or-to-heat studios, temporary spaces, bedrooms with no sound privacy, neighbor complaints, windowless bedrooms, broken toilets, and moldy showers. It is a history of extraordinary resourcefulness, vibrant community, abundant meals, creative innovation, all-night discussions, restless experimentation, collective effort, unbelievably gorgeous performances, and sublime happiness: 1800SF, 848, Blake Street Hawkeyes, CELLspace, Chez Bushwick, Club Foot, the Garage, Highways, Hub14, K77 Studio, the downstairs space at Performance Space 122, Performance Works NW, Pieter, the Sawtooth Building on Eighth Street, Studio 4, Studio 210, Sugar Shack.

In *The Gentrification of the Mind* (2012), Sarah Schulman complicates the perspective that white or college-educated artists and queers moving into and creating spaces in predominantly poor, Black, Brown, immigrant, and "failed" neighborhoods is a settler-colonial move, a gentrifying move, arguing that it is the result of forced migration, a tactic of economic and social refugees. Schulman points out that it is generally not the artists who create new restaurants or shops, gentrifying and segregating the economies and ecologies of a neighborhood. The standard framing is that white bohemians are on the front line of gentrification. White artists can exoticize and romanticize a low-income neighborhood as if they hadn't been privileged from birth by a racial real-estate hierarchy that significantly contributes to the racialized inequity that undermines social solidarity and democracy. Broke artists, collectivist anarchists, freaks from the economic and queer margins, refugees from homophobic and suffocating small towns and suburbs, dancers surviving on restaurant or sex work illegally repurpose abandoned commercial buildings to make hybrid live-work spaces where art and community can flourish in what author and poet Hakim Bey aspirationally refers to as "temporary autonomous zones." Most artists are gentrified out of these neighborhoods within one or two generations. Marginalized in our own ways, we rarely buy property and are brutally forced out to search for the next "affordable" area, ever farther from the culturally rich centers we helped to constellate. Photographer Janet Delaney notes, "Most of the artists that I ever interacted with were on the street, getting to know their community, working politically as well as doing their own artwork. Their presence may make an area seem more accessible to outsiders. But developers are gentrifiers, government zoning laws have aided gentrification, people with money who can manipulate the market are the ones who create and benefit from gentrification." Are dancers precarious workers and economic migrants, or are we gentrifiers and neoliberal settlers? Yes, no, but, and...

A history of dance is a history of sex work.

In the nineteenth century, skirt dancers flashed their legs to a predominantly male audience in cabaret and burlesque theaters. Loïe Fuller, an innovator of costuming, dance, and theatrical lighting, emerged from this context yet has been elevated as a pioneer of modern dance without the stain that marked her contemporaries. From approximately 1850 to 1909, when Nijinsky arrived in

Paris, male ballet dancers were not featured on European or US stages. The female dancer, en travesti, played male roles without skirts to cover her legs. Clad only in tights, her legs subtly scandalized and titillated her bourgeois male audience. Then there are the stories of female dancers from the Paris Opera mingling with the audience after the performance, especially with the wealthier male donors who subsidized the production. Close observers identify these encounters as prostitution and even sexual coercion. The dancer's body and the choreographed performance are archives of erotic embodiment, prurient entertainment, the colonial gaze, and puritanical framing.

In my extended community in the 1980s and early 1990s, sex-positive feminists and gay dancers responded to the trauma of AIDS by connecting with the erotic-massage school Body Electric as part of a movement reclaiming and contemporizing archetypes of the sacred prostitute and sexual healer. And so many women artists found part-time work at the Lusty Lady, one of the few strip clubs where customers could not touch the dancers, an aspect of the job that attracted many feminist-identified sex workers but promised lower pay until a union was formed and the business became a co-op.

At least one person in every collaborative or group I've produced in the past twenty-five years has engaged in sex work to help pay for essentials like rent and food and the costs associated with dancing, including classes and body care. I can't count how many friends and collaborators, most with college degrees, did sex work to be able to afford the double "privileges" of being an artist and living in the Bay Area. Sex work has almost been a rite of passage for gay male artists in San Francisco. Sex work offers a flexibility amenable to project-based artists, and it brings in more pay than food service, teaching, or dancing in theaters. Extensive skills are needed to avoid the racial, class, and gender antagonisms of a mostly male clientele. Almost every artist I know who has done sex work wanted to quit months or years before they finally did. It has an emotional and psychic cost that is made worse by its illegality.

Religious communities throughout history have charged dancers with inciting lust and have instituted dancing bans. Indigenous cultures have endured ruthless antidance laws. The critique of Bill T. Jones's Tony-award-winning *Fela* (2008) as being too sexual repeated a trope of shaming that has been used against dance for centuries, especially Black and Indigenous dance, such as pelvis-centered African-diasporic dances but also flamenco, salsa, and the tarantella. "Hence my discomfort," reported a white *New York Times* theater critic. "The presentation of African culture as a feast of exotic pageantry has the potential, at least, to reinforce stereotypes of African people as primitive and unsophisticated, albeit endowed with astounding aptitudes for song and dance.... And the way the dancers weave in and out of the audience repeatedly seems ingratiating, a sort of seduction that almost sexualizes the performers." Oh, there is so much decolonizing of dance and sex that we still have to do! *Fela*'s exposed bodies and vibrant dancing proposed a reconsideration of the cultural and healing roles of erotic dance.

German theater director René Pollesch is credited with saying that contemporary dance is softcore for the bourgeoisie. And it is true that legions of productions, including my own, stage nude and nearly nude dancers, often in physical contact or proximity, and produce images that portray the erotic or sexual—and not only in small and underfunded theaters but in large state-funded theaters and festivals. Recalling Barbara Ehrenreich's *Dancing in the Streets*, which explores how various religious doctrines have forbidden and even led to the criminalization of dancing, performance artist Philip Huang writes, "Sexual, tranced, communal dance around fires was lost to Christianity, colonialism, and the rise of the individual. Dance was a threatening act BECAUSE it was sexual.

Putting ritual dance onstage contains it, turns it even more lurid, a peepshow. We went from everyone being a ritual participant to nearly everyone being a peeper."

Here are a few snapshots from the past twenty years (names changed because sex-work stigma is real): Jaime, with a bachelor's degree from the University of California, Santa Cruz, as well as professional experience in both contemporary dance and Mexican *folklórico*, worked weekly as a go-go dancer in gay clubs, wearing a jockstrap in one bar and dancing naked in a plexiglass-enclosed shower in another. Working in contemporary dance and performance as circus artists, Jasmine and Trina each started stripping professionally at sixteen. By eighteen, Trina looked back at her stripping days as a phase of her youth, while Jasmine had transitioned to providing a full-service girlfriend experience. An undocumented artist living in the United States since she was a teenager, Jasmine had ongoing transactional relationships with three different men for five years. In satisfying their Asian fetish, they covered her rent, expensive circus training, and basic living expenses. My queer sister Dana trained with a legendary professional dominatrix, first assisting her and then working with her own clients. When Raymond was broke, he went to a Tenderloin bar frequented by trans women, cross-dressers, and their admirers. In full drag, she offered straight men the opportunity to suck Black dick. Jen transitioned from happy-ending massage in a local woman-run business to full-service prostitution when she realized that she could reduce her sex work to less than a month per year. To supplement her dance income from teaching and performing in a company, she would travel to Southern California to work seven to ten days in a row, seeing multiple clients daily. Curt has performed a story in which he tears pages from a hotel room's Gideon Bible, dropping them onto his bound client in a ritual exorcism of Christian sex shame. Kiara used her experience as a queer Black sex worker to reframe her relationship to me and other white male artists who hire or produce Black artists. She said that she related to me as a hooker relates to a john and that this indicated not only the structural inequity of the relationship but also its potential for her agency.

A history of dance is a history of embodiment.

Dance histories are written and rewritten not in books but in rehearsal, practice, party, and performance. If you go to the arts section of any bookstore, there will be no subsection within it smaller than that for dance. And you will have to dance to see it: the dance section choreographs the reader to get down on the ground to the bottom shelf or gaze upward, reaching overhead to the top shelf. Dance history hardly exists in written form. Maybe this lack of books and easy access to them has protected the embodied histories of dance.

The dance archive is more likely to live and die on YouTube, TikTok, Vimeo, Douyin, and Wikipedia—in apps, sites, and other dance-sharing platforms and technologies. Dance drives the video-sharing industry. The kids are learning to dance online. Ultimately, though, the archive lives in the bodies of dancers. The dance archive survives and transforms through embodied transmission, from dancer to dancer, teacher to student, studio to studio. My memory and body contain a living, growing archive that will not die when I do.

As a young artist, my reading focused on political and experimental theater, especially the Living Theater. I coveted the writings of Julian Beck and Judith Malina and the photos and stories of Paradise Now, the collective ensemble and sexual-liberation performance born of nonviolent anarchist politics. After immersing myself in the Living, I read about Antonin Artaud, Eugenio Barba, Bread and Puppet Theater, Joseph Chaikin,

Richard Foreman, Gardzienice, Jerzy Grotowski, Tadeusz Kantor, Richard Schechner, and the Wooster Group. While this reflects a (mostly) white-dude canon, it also points to how theater history was so much better documented and more accessible to a young left-leaning autodidact embarking on a career in live performance in the late seventies and early eighties. And so it's no surprise that my first full-length solo performance, *Saliva*, was inspired not by a dancer but by Karen Finley, a writer, theater maker, and performance artist.

Who populates my body's archive? From Montréal, I assimilated the influence of the women's improvisation collective Carbone 14; Catpoto; a young Marie Chouinard; Margie Gillis, who showed me that no amount of emotion was too much to express through dancing; Le Groupe Nouvelle Aire; Andrew Harwood; Jo Lechay; and Mime Omnibus. The improvisers who inspire my dancing body include Ishmael Houston-Jones; Lucas Hoving, who, with cellist Gwendolyn Watson, modeled a technical rigor that continues to shape my improvised performances; Mangrove; Sara Shelton Mann and Terry Sendgraff, who created a home for me in their studios and their hearts, which were often indistinguishable; Ed Mock and Akira Kasai, who cleared a path for me in which anything could happen—a nearly boundaryless space where artistic disciplines and genres were irrelevant and where camp humor and deep abstraction were siblings. In collaboration, my body and consciousness have been altered by experiences in performance with multitudes of dancers, musicians, and artists. I had a special familial and creative relationship with Jules Beckman, Jess Curtis, and Norman Rutherford (of Contraband), which endured for many years. For nearly a decade, my dance and improvisation were embedded within the Turbulence collaborative, and these practices of queer kinship, theatrical deconstruction, and rejection of disciplinary or dramaturgical coherence still feel fresh in my body, teaching, and choreography. I've also enjoyed wild and pleasurable relationships with Jassem Hindi and Houston-Jones, who have been liberating partners in improvised performance. Guillermo Gomez-Peña dynamically recited a poetic text while I coated my legs in blood donated by the audience to prepare me for ritualized dancing. Essex Hemphill sat on my bed while we rewrote each other's poems. Faustin Linyekula shocked students by walking out of our workshop, the Political Body, while I explained that, no, I wouldn't be going after him, since we had agreed that we didn't have to present a unified front. Peaches and I staged an extraordinary concert in Vienna attended by more than two thousand people. Meg Stuart brought a chicken from the grocery store onstage, handing it to me as we improvised with others in *Auf den Tisch*. Gerald Casel shared healing dances with me on a beach and at a farm. J Jha and I traded texts outside Homeland Security. And with Annie Danger and one hundred witches, I hexed City Hall to develop policies of abolition, reparations, housing, and sanctuary.

A history of dance is a history of bodily transformation.

Every dancer has a body project, whether intentional, externally imposed, neurotically compliant, or clearly designed. Weight loss. Turn out. Increased flexibility. Muscle mass. Techniques for balancing, spinning, jumping, landing. Physical ideals and comparisons. Body shame and dysmorphia. Body honoring and celebration. Fetishization and inadequacy. Few dancers can relax in the identity of enough: good enough, strong enough, thin enough. A conflict between the spectacle and the somatic: "How do I look?" versus "How do I feel?" Despite the recent integration of somatic, feminist, antiracist, and healing practices into ballet and contemporary dance training, the body shaming of women dancers persists and has only intensified thanks to Insta filters and TikTok. The mirror is everywhere, and the reflection is a lie.

One of my teachers didn't have a period for several years while training and dancing with notable professional companies in New York. It's extraordinary when you think about it—the anorexia and the stress deactivated her body's attunement to the movement of the ocean and planets. Repetitive movement gestures and movement patterns strengthen but ultimately weaken the body. The body works too hard and pays for it later, rehearses when tired and performs while injured, attempts difficult movements before it is ready. Cartilage wears and tears. Bones grind. Pain sears. The dancer accommodates limited mobility and chronic pain. It leads to years of care practices for anyone who can afford them, from yoga and bodywork to surgery, physical therapy, cortisone shots, and artificial joints.

A brief list of legendary dance artists with one or two hip replacements: Anne Bluethenthal, choreographer and founder of Skywatchers, a company of artists working in between dance, social/relational practices, activism, healing, and public ritual in San Francisco's Tenderloin neighborhood; Jess Curtis, choreographer, artist, director of Gravity, former dancer with Mann's Contraband, and emerging expert in the field of access services; Dieter Heitkamp, cofounder of Berlin's Tanzfabrik, a pioneering contact-improvisation teacher–organizer–performer in Germany and longtime professor of dance education at the University for Music and Performing Arts in Frankfurt am Main, Germany; Monique Jenkinson, aka Fauxnique, dancer, drag artist, and author, known for being the first faux queen to win Miss Trannyshack, a major drag title in San Francisco's 1990s queer underground; Krissy Keefer, cofounder of the feminist dance companies Wallflower Order and the Dance Brigade, artistic director of the vibrant dance venue Dance Mission, and cofounder of the feminist-led after-school dance-and-drumming program Grrl Brigade; Maurya Kerr, choreographer of tinypistol who was forced into early ballet retirement after eight years with Lines Ballet and three hip replacements in six years but is still dancing; Louise Lecavalier, fierce dancer best known for her performances with Montréal's La La La Human Steps, choreographed by Édouard Lock, and internationally recognized as an innovative, gender-bending diva of postmodern dance (most barrel rolls ever?); Sara Shelton Mann, founder and choreographer of Contraband and highly influential Bay Area dance teacher and researcher working at the intersections of healing, transpersonal experience, dance, improvisation, consciousness, and presence; Elizabeth Roxas-Dobrish, former Ailey dancer and teacher who dared to dance *Revelations* with the company after a total hip replacement. Is this how these dancers want to be known, to be archived? Aren't the stories of their dancing, decades of dancing, more important than the impact of that dancing, the price of that dancing?

A history of dance is a history of spirals, rituals, and circles.

Sometime in the 1980s, at a ritual protest, I experienced my first spiral dance. It was most likely an antiwar or antinuclear-weapons protest. Within the nonviolent direct-action community was a well-networked community of anarchist, feminist witches called Reclaiming, many living in collective houses in the Bay Area. The spiral dance, as I learned it from Reclaiming, begins with everyone holding hands in a circle. The leader lets go of the person to their left and begins to walk slowly counterclockwise along the inner curve of the circle. Usually, there is drumming and a repeating chant. Once the entire group is spiraling inward, the leader switches direction and begins to walk clockwise, leading folks to spiral outward and face the dancers who are still spiraling inward. As the dance continues, every dancer comes face to face, however briefly, with every other dancer. Queer artist and witch Jack Davis told me, "You get to see everyone who is there face to face, and I can feel the energy rising as we spiral and sing and see each other." I know no other circle-dance choreography that can move mass groups and retain this person-to-person intimacy. For Reclaiming, the goal is to raise energy and then focus it as healing for political change. A spell or magic involves symbolic activity in one realm to influence another.

Reclaiming calls the spiral dance a traditional dance, although its most recorded tradition is linked to *The Spiral Dance*, an iconic text of the Euro pagan and neopagan movements. The book, first published in 1979, was written by ecofeminist author, activist, and teacher Starhawk, a founding member of Reclaiming and my neighbor in San Francisco. The spiral dance is an annual ritual marking Samhain, or Halloween, a festival of death and rebirth temporally linked to the end of the harvest season in the Northern Hemisphere. At this Samhain ritual, the community is invited to visit with the beloved dead before joining a massive circle with as many as a thousand people, dancing the spiral in a celebration of life and as a spell to help manifest our visions for the next year.

Is the dance ancient or New Age? Is it traditional or postcolonial? Is the spiral dance a rooted practice or a practice that, like the diasporic settlers who "reclaimed" it, floats. I call it the oldest dance I know, even though I have little historical data to support that claim. Many cultures practice or have practiced a dance of walking in a spiral. I once witnessed a quick-stepping spiral dance, much like that of Reclaiming, by Cuban dancers enacting an embodiment of both Yoruban deities and enslaved peoples. And I have read about dancers from the Wyandotte Nation (Oklahoma) whose snake dance involves a line of dancers moving into a tight spiral and then shifting direction to unwind.

I can't remember the first time I saw a Native-led round dance or the first time I danced in one. It was an early choreographic influence that demonstrated how dancing can create and nurture community. A staple at powwows across Turtle Island, particularly in the United States and Canada, the most common round dance involves a repeating two-step movement timed with drumming. With distinct regional and tribal styles of drumming and footwork and particular intentions and reasons to dance, there are infinite variations of NDN[1] dances that circle. Sometimes the host of the round dance will invite everyone to join, regardless of tribal identity or cultural familiarity. Originating with the Plains Indians, the round dance has survived colonial erasure, has been adopted as a universal practice among Turtle Island tribal and intertribal gatherings, and more recently has become a practice of ritualized civil disobedience for Indigenous activists.

I first witnessed NDN activists round dancing in a 2012 YouTube video of Idle No More crowding a shopping mall in Western Canada. Idle No More and other Native and First Nation communities have since staged hundreds of flash-mob round dances across Turtle Island in nontraditional contexts, including shopping malls, pipeline-construction sites, and government buildings and during street protests. These dances serve complex functions, raising awareness about Indigenous struggles and culture; building solidarity and nurturing resistance; and healing multigenerational trauma through cultural visibility that affirms a role for prayer, ritual, and dancing.

Plains dancers move clockwise to the left, following the sun, which is the directional choreography practiced by many Native American tribes. I was at a workshop led by a few California Natives who said they had only recently learned that their ancestors had danced the circle to the right, with the center, or fire, closer to the left or heart side of the body. Traditions change. Genocidal settler colonialism attempted to destroy NDN dancing, and a new generation of Indigenous "Californians" has begun to unwind the circle, complicate the tradition, and reclaim the dance.

1 NDN: Indian, Native, First Nations (Canada), Indigenous, aboriginal, autochthonous. Each of these terms might be appropriate in one context or another, for one community or another. Sometimes, these terms are used interchangeably, as I use them, and other times, they have very particular meanings and importance where it would be inappropriate to mix them. I am using NDN, among other terms, because I recently read Billy-Ray Belcourt's gorgeous memoir, *A History of My Brief Body*, where he uses NDN throughout. Belcourt is a queer NDN writer and scholar from the Driftpile Cree Nation (Alberta, Canada).

Many dance classes are choreographed in lines or grids, with everyone facing toward the teacher or choreographer and perhaps a mirror. In contact-improv spaces and experimental-dance contexts, dancers have gathered in circles for decades, usually to begin and end a class and then practice in a decentered or decentralized choreography responding to the teacher's prompts for personal or collective research. Gathering in a circle in the dance studio is much more common today than forty years ago. The influence of Indigenous cultural practices on American mainstream cultures might be difficult to track systematically, but it cannot be overstated. Hippie, post-hippie, and countercultural movements are obvious sites of Indigenous influence and appropriation. But even in their absence or extremely diluted forms, Indigenous practices have been influential to the artists who have deliberately sought to undermine normative culture. Where better could we look for perspectives on decolonization than Black and Indigenous culture? In circles, no one's position is more valued or visible than anyone else's, and each person can be heard by everyone else.

Observing circular, spiral, and infinite movement in our bodies, in nature, in the galactic and more-than-human bodies around us, we learn not only easy and efficient movement but also concrete proposals for a new kind of seeing, listening, conceptualizing, planning, and social organizing.

+++

And as we drop deeper into these proposals, maybe we'll notice that time has passed and that we've changed, that the ground underneath us is marked by collective movement and that our relationships with one another, however precarious and fragile, are more easily held when dancing together than when not.

Bring your folks, that would be us,
the beyond bodied.
—Alexis Pauline Gumbs[1]

At a recent performance choreographed by Meg Stuart at the Hammer Museum in Los Angeles, dancer Varinia Canto Vila made history.[2] It wasn't the first performance in the galleries of a museum or the first time a South American dancer performed in North America. Rather, it was a movement that Canto Vila made—a single, fully embodied gesture—that caused me to recognize the moment as distinctly historic. Spread across the floor, Canto Vila moved in a nonambulatory crawl, frenetically still—a striving expressed as internally driven. The contradictory vectors of this movement seemingly reached outward from an overexposed armpit toward a vanishing finish line, reverberating in a face that contorted without strain. The movement barely went anywhere; the movement seemed to go everywhere. As I mimetically interpolated this into my own body, I felt the illogic of its kinesthesia, the ways in which it couldn't fit my body, my projection or recognition of movement; indeed, it couldn't fit into my understanding of a human body. My inability to integrate what was immediately foreign to me felt both strange and familiar to my experience as a spectator of dance. But this time, what was unresolved articulated into the debris of a thought: *This is the first time in history that anyone has ever done that movement.*

1 Alexis Pauline Gumbs, *Dub: Finding Ceremony* (Durham, NC: Duke University Press, 2020), 237.

2 Meg Stuart and Varinia Canto Vila performed *confirm humanity* from March 8 to 13, 2022, as part of the exhibition *Lifes*, Hammer Museum, Los Angeles, February 16–May 8, 2022.

Of course, I don't know, will never know, if that's true—if any movement has ever occurred for the first time or if every movement occurs for the first time. But that moment compelled me to consider the possibility that a new movement could emerge. If so, from where? How? Why not before? What would this new movement require to become truly unlike any movement ever performed before, and what, if anything, could a completely novel movement *do*? In light of these thoughts, refracting from the body I witnessed writhing while barely moving, dance felt fundamentally like both a contradiction and a proposition, a rendering of what bodies could be through a lens of becoming.

In that frame, the history of dance seemed less a matter of what happened and more about what could have happened. The history of dance could be coextensive if not synonymous with the history of possible bodies.

Anatomically and biologically, there's little daylight between the body of Canto Vila and that of a prehistorical human or a human from the third or tenth or twenty-first century. Everything manifested in that bizarre moment of embodied history/making was always possible for a person to do. The dance that Canto Vila performed, horizontally splayed, hardly moving but seemingly caught within an attempt to move regardless, has existed in its potentiality for eons; one could say it was always available but immanently, intimately, asymptotically unreachable. But if it was always already physically possible to perform this movement, why did I feel certain that it had never happened on this Earth before?

Maybe a dance is like an idea whose time has come.
—Wesley Brown[3]

One reading might say that this movement was always a potentiality but never actually possible because ideology choreographs us. By this interpretation, culture writes the body and, therefore, what a body can possibly be and do. A body from the third century could not perform Canto Vila's movement because an ideology from that time would never permit, instruct, or construct a body to perform it. From this perspective, there's no escape from history and the ideologies that are written using our bodies, only occasional subversive acts of flight that, if we're lucky, will be reinscribed into "the history" of bodies or, if not, will likely be forgotten.

Another perspective comes to us from *The Embodied Mind* (1992), in which Francisco J. Varela, Eleanor Rosch, and Evan Thompson argue that in early development, it is the embryo's movement that creates and structures thought, not the other way around.[4] The embryo moves, creating the neural pathways that formulate the structures and reasons for movement and the feelings associated with those movements or the feelings of not being able to fulfill or perform those movements. In the thought/movement fold, movement is always a beat ahead, which is perhaps why a new movement can't be solely prethought and why what we might call a new movement is literally unimaginable.

3 Wesley Brown, *Tragic Magic* (San Francisco: McSweeney's, 2021), 127.

4 Francisco J. Varela, Eleanor Rosch, and Evan Thompson, *The Embodied Mind: Cognitive Science and Human Experience* (Cambridge, MA: MIT Press, 1992).

(But much of history is unwritten.
Remember this.)
—N. K. Jemisin[5]

If history is the appearance of the new inscribed into the known, what's potentially fascinating about a history of dance is that bodies and their movements generally seem to resist such inscription. The history of moving bodies is a history that plays sleights of hand with presence and disappearance. The moment Canto Vila performed that unplaceable movement, the lineages that had carried her body there, all the folks that had joined together to make that movement arrive in that moment, were hidden by the very same body. That gathering of generations—which nonetheless appeared singular and stirringly new—simultaneously escaped capture, stubbornly retaining its status as unknown. The history of dance is littered with such unknown movements, unknown dancers, and unknown dances; the history of dance is mostly unknown. The history of dance might be written about, but it is not written. It is uttered—by which I mean it operates with the rare privileges of its own poor sign economy. Dance says, but what it says is seldom what's heard. Indeed, to "understand" or "get" a dance hardly, if ever, means that what's gotten equals what was served—this is the irregular geometry of a performance's unwritten contract.

5 N. K. Jemisin, *The Fifth Season* (New York: Orbit, 2015), 3.

Uttering—an act that simultaneously produces and evades meaning—is a dancing body's modus operandi, or perhaps her unshakable best frenemy, one that also produces while it evades history. It seems that utterance—rather than the symbolic order of writing or oration—isn't entirely conducive to the discipline of history, or better still, with such utterings, a dancing body might propose other ways for us to understand what history could be.

All origins are arbitrary. This is not to say that they are not also nurturing, but they are essentially coercive and indifferent.
—Dionne Brand[6]

History, she say, is queens and kings and wars and treaties, inventions, monuments to progress, and moments of rupture; the victors, they tell us, write the history. But a fold ahead of the queen—before she declares war, signs treaties, or seals the deeds to sell other bodies, before she dies and a new successor is named, before any of that—is her body. Before the fates of bodies deciding, or the fates of bodies decided upon, are their bodies; before the history of bodies can be written is the body, which is to say, the virtual, spiritual, mythological, physical, and extraphysical manifestation of an idea we call "body." The history of dance is the history of utterances and reutterances of what that idea could be. That history is rarely, barely written; and to try and write it would seem counter to its very project.

Yet sometimes we try. Dance-history writing bounces along in entangled movements from firsthand testimonials of emerging scenes (think *Paris Is Burning*) to storied genealogies espousing singular origins (think twerking).

Claimed by some to have originated at the 2013 MTV Music Video Awards, when it was performed by Miley, or else from a combination of the dances known as the jerk and the twist in North America in the 1960s, or else from New Orleans bounce in the 1980s, or else from the Mapouka dance from Côte d'Ivoire centuries ago, twerking is one of

6 Dionne Brand, *A Map to the Door of No Return: Notes to Belonging* (New York: Penguin Random House, 2023), 64.

the unnecessarily contested sites that emerge from the "coercive and indifferent" tendencies of origin stories. Twerking can be said to be a highly sexualized, profane dance, a religiously devotional dance, or a tribal dance that celebrates family gatherings in communal acts of joy. What these stories have in common, regardless of their veracity, is that they tend to reveal more about their authors than about dance itself, invoking notions of authenticity and theft that resituate dance within the very object status it goes—literally—to great pains to try and escape. Dances like Canto Vila's, avoid being posited within a history of dance that would like to plot the points that led to their emergence.

Surely predominant is the version of dance history that, like an archive of property deeds to a given address, says who owned what and when. But dance isn't property any more than bodies are, and when it is, we have no choice but to demand abolition.

the ownership of movement,
abolish
the conflation of authorship and ownership,
abolish
an ensemble of bodies as the property
of a single author,
abolish
the myth of a single author,
abolish
a history that moves to uphold any
of the above
abolish

I don't own the movements this body has performed, even if I (the we that I be) may have uttered them many times. That's my relationship to this body, which has many boundaries but is not mine. That's my experience of this location, where many other bodies gather, in din and occasional harmony, to form a me that belongs to no one, least of all me.[7]

When I move this body, I summon (though I cannot always control) the bodies I want to move through. I choose which bodies I wish to call in (though not always; some bodies haunt mine). Some bodies don't leave, even when I've asked them to; some bodies won't come back, no matter how many times I call them. My body accumulates and, sure, forgets but never as much as I think it might. I don't belong to the story history likes to tell, the one where it articulates its own memory of itself.

I belong to a different kind of history, the kind that believes origins, families, and identities articulate a making and unmaking as we move along. I bumble and blur through the myriad of ways I've been choreographed—by dance and otherwise—hardly able to tell the choreographies and choreographers of my body apart. That blur means that the movements of one dance might be rechoreographed by the qualities of another; that a repertory that may exist on video still smudges when, years later, it reenters my body, changed by aging and new experience; or that a choreography I've performed many times continues to repeat,

7 Dramaturge Elaine Carberry, in conversation with the author, October 31, 2021.

in its underlying sense and logics and rhythms, long after the last time I think I've performed it. That blur means that, unlike the version of a history that stands on a land it has called its own, the body records history somewhat closer to the way history actually is—as fungible, inherently fallible, with neither telos nor origin, written and rewritten in and by the same material, the same body, that makes that history, even as it sometimes struggles to remember its own name.

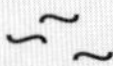

I don't believe in history (or at least the story it tells itself), and despite years of working as a choreographer, I still don't know what dance is. Which is also to say, I don't know what isn't dance. And because of this, when I try and reflect on the history of dance, the question only seems to hot-potato back onto itself: *What's the dance of history?*

When does one decide to stop looking to the past and instead conceive of a new order?
—Saidiya Hartman[8]

The dance of history could be frontal, linear, cyclical, or entropic. It could be an endless rehearsal, repeating again and again with a difference, trying to get its movements just right. It could be an ongoing improvisational jam, without aim, or an expertly virtuosic display of well-structured human prowess. It could be a meandering, stumbling dance through the dark, murmuring and stuttering as it runs into the invisible pieces of its own set design, or a dance of grand narratives of progress and crises, with a fateful conclusion just before the curtain falls. The dance of history could be a chorus of growing, accelerating bodies moving in concert or in chaos, a tight-knit company wherein kin dance together, or a mass of bodies randomly thrown into the same space, individualized and individuated. This dance could be dramaturgically crafted, with a sense of narrative direction and purpose, or smooth and flat, ongoing and durational, indifferent to beginnings, middles, and ends.

I don't believe in history, and I don't know what dance is. And yet I'll admit there's a compelling story there. The story goes: mating rituals, labor rituals, non- or preverbal religious and spiritual rituals, uncodified at first, developing a grammar, contexts, mythologies, symbolic, semiotic, and sensed meanings. It goes from simple to complex, communal to formal. It goes from nothing to something, built up and then mechanized, becoming a technology that produced the idea of the body as much as it was

8 Saidiya Hartman, *Lose Your Mother: A Journey along the Atlantic Slave Route* (New York: Farrar, Straus and Giroux, 2008), 100.

produced by bodies, instituted and eventually institutionalized, celebrated then memorialized; it goes from free play to language, repeatable and then canonized. It goes from communing with spirits and deities to communing with others, to sharing experience-objects, to objectifying itself, to dealing with the problems of its objectified status, and back to communing with spirits. The story goes from the organization of movement in time and space to developing a methodology for working with the movement of bodies, nonbodies, and beyond, to becoming a politic, a series of tools with which to proceed in any medium, that we might nevertheless still call *choreography*. It goes from dealing with the body as nature to an extension of nature; to a moldable, docile, cultured being; to a laboratory for a moldable society, a raw material confronting its own acceleration, dematerialization, and disappearance. It goes from real to artificial, to virtual, to prototyping a real we might only begin to imagine. The compelling story accumulates, and as it does, it folds and repeats.

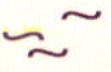

While one fold told us that we have individual bodies (an idea that has been particularly helpful to capitalization and exploitation), another repeatedly uttered otherwise. She say, the body is plastic, nonsingular, individual as it is communal. Movement courses through it—the movement of thoughts, experiences, and images, a feedback loop that can never be closed between inside out and outside in. Internal movements in dialogue with external environments and outward-facing needs and drives. If there is a history of dance, it is as much a history of becoming as it is one of undoing, a movement that weaves as it unravels.

To move the body within and through the world is to articulate both the specificity and the location in which that body exists as much as it is to propose a body that may not yet be *us*. To watch a body moving is to interpolate that potential body, an act of kinesthetic sympathy projected inward. When we say a dance is *good*, it may mean that this foreign body has been accepted protogenetically by our body; to say it is *bad* may mean to reject it, to say this is not ours, not us, not our body, it has not moved a me to a we, or perhaps it's a we that has already been and is no longer needed in order to move—perhaps it is his or hers or theirs but is not *our* potential body.

And what or who would this we be? I don't know who we think we are, but I know how dance has led me to encounter—again and again—so many we's I want to be.

≈~

As I imagine the dance of history coursing through us, I picture a troupe with no director and no repertory, that doesn't assume too much about where it's from, certainly not where it's going. Bound by the fault lines of our differences, by the common ways we undo what we thought we knew, the ways we tend to weave our strands back together, and how we serve them, despite it all, anew. So disbanded that we've come together, a tribe without cohesions, a motley neighborhood of din. In the dance of history I imagine, we dance to imagine, collectively, an ahistorical future. We dance to conjure disassembly. We disassemble by communing, commune by gathering, gather by moving over and making room, making room so we can know: *now we that too*.

Don't get it twisted: We is deeply in love with our past, our folks, 'cause they's us too, coursing through and through. The dance of history we imagine don't confuse ancestors for predecessors. Our ancestry ain't history but is presence. We is a project of listening, paying attention to how we can cohere and disassemble better and better as more ancestors arrive, *make room!* 'Cuz we prefer dissonance to erasure. And our dance of history includes the movement of future generations, some so young they may not yet speak words—why would history not claim what they got to say too?

We have neither the time nor privilege nor belief in permanence to want to build or protect a territory, to distinguish what's important from what's not; it's all too proximal and intimate to objectify.

Our we ain't interested in what's old or what's current. Our we is interested in *the current*, where and how it's moving, what feeds it and what hinders it, and yeah, we include obstacles as part of our history too.

~ ~ ~

Of late, some of the biggest stones standing in our current have been distance, forces of separation, illness, violence, mass death, the dangers of gathering our bodies close with strangers to experience things together.

As I write this at the end of 2022, it's hard not to reflect on these past couple of years, when our dance of history seemed to race toward immobilities choreographed by a pandemic. Illness often immobilizes the body, at least outwardly; internally, there's usually a different story, as the body's defenses spring into motion. These past years, while our collective body fought off illness, our defenses sprang into action.

One major defense that has choreographed our immobility of late has been fear. Borders and edicts reinforced by fear, including the defensive auto-immune ones that claim to keep *us* (the overdetermined "us") healthy by keeping others out, have sought to immobilize our body. The ever-persistent practice of incarceration—keeping *us* safe by keeping others confined—increasingly immobilizes our body. The interfaces that we've been using to carry out our remote work, rehearsing a frontal, mediated relationship to the world, have attempted to immobilize our body. We've been up against some paralyzing shit these days. But still we move, and resistance to movement is part of our dance history too.

So how do we continue to move through, with, and against forces of immobility? I learn from Canto Vila, hurtling through a sprawl so wide and so low that it rendered itself into a catapulted grounding, self-confined but far from inert, moving within its arrest. I learn from the ways that moment embodied the double meaning of *inertia*—referring to a body both at rest and in motion—and from practicing the two as potentially noncontradictory. But I also learn from two other dances—one liberatory and the other horrifically fatal—dances that history might hardly call such.

In 1849, after enduring thirty-three years in slavery, Henry Box Brown shipped himself by post in a box—two-by-three feet in size—from a plantation in Virginia to freedom in Philadelphia. That dance, confined but vaulted into motion, across state lines that demarcated his body's status as property or free, moved from the objectification of his body to its liberation via a clever, extra-objectification in drag as parcel. Once free, Brown went on to perform vaudeville reenactments of this feat, seeming to echo the preternatural performativity of his high-stakes act as a potential catalyst to alter both circumstance and conscience.

In considering Brown's propelled immobility, perhaps whether the body moves or not is less important than what its moving or not moves. Perhaps the confinement imposed by borders that immobilize us can be rendered performative too, crossed by fugitive choreographies that restage immobility. And still, we move.

The second dance calls to me from an opposing direction—one that leads to not freedom but mortal harm. In 2015, the Baltimore Police arrested Freddie Carlos Gray Jr., aka Freddie Gray, for possession of a switchblade—which it was legal for him to have. The officers loaded Gray into the back of a police van and gave him a "rough ride"—in which a person in handcuffs is not given a seatbelt and is tossed about by excessively violent or erratic driving. All the officers involved were, unsurprisingly, acquitted. Gray fell into a coma and later died.

Why evoke Gray's body in a meditation on dance and history? Uncomfortable as it might be—not least for me—to ask for a consideration of that horrific incident and so many others like it, both known and unknown to history as dance, I also think it might lend some perspective.

Dancing is not an endorsement of violence but of course it is.
—Simone White[9]

Dance can abstract a body, and so can violence. The vectors that constitute these voluntary and involuntary pathways create their own forms of movement. The violence of confinement—the project to render a body immobile, which is to say nonliving, or mobile only for certain aims, such as involuntary labor or juridically sanctioned punishment—could be said to be quintessentially antidance. And dance has been said to be quintessentially liberatory. But that particular abstraction of the body we call dance is not always voluntary and not always nonviolent.

The dance of death we call violence, equal parts cult and cultural tradition, choreographed by states of fear and desires to subdue certain bodies while emboldening others—is no less a dance because it's unappealing and ugly. This dance has its own techniques and traditions, its own rehearsals and performances. If we allow it to, this dance can remind us that dance, too, can be base, profane, and lethal; that dance has nothing whatsoever to do with liberation or care or with the subtle negotiations between consenting bodies, not exclusively or even with autonomy or free will. Dance can require docile bodies to do its work, as much as its work can render bodies docile. It can motivate and immobilize, it can be a doing and a being done to, made by artists and uni(n)formed villains alike. Dance is not good, dance is not warm; dance is not ours. Which is to say, we may need to fight for dance.

9 Simone White, *or, on being the other woman* (Durham, NC: Duke University Press, 2022), 48.

The score: Manifest a dance integral to the
sympoiesis of bodies, a dance that helps us
imagine, perhaps become, the bodies we
have yet to be.[10] Without flattening our we into
a singularity. Recognizing, even calling in the
dances that run counter to our pursuit,
lending our bodies to this friction. Recognizing
that these dances don't call themselves
such. Recognizing that, like it or not, they's
our history too.

10 Theorist Donna Haraway coined the term *sympoiesis* in reference to "complex, dynamic, responsive, situated, historical systems," deriving it from the ancient Greek *sún* ("with, together") and *poíēsis* ("creation, production"), meaning "making-with" or "becoming-with." Donna Haraway, *Staying with the Trouble: Making Kin in the Chthulucene* (Durham, NC: Duke University Press, 2016), 58.

En route to Stockholm recently, one in a group of friends asked aloud how Stockholm syndrome got its name. The term was coined in the 1970s after hostages taken in a Swedish bank heist refused to testify against their captors and instead helped raise funds for their criminal defense. *Stockholm syndrome* is usually employed to shame someone for their refusal to wish harm on those who have caused them harm. "Sounds like abolition," said one friend. "Stockholm syndrome—that's what we do."

A dance with Stockholm syndrome might help us down this current. A dance that calls in rather than calls out. A dance that calls in even those bodies and practices that might be considered most detestable, most cruel, most violent. They are, like it or not, our bodies too. And what happens, I wonder, when we relinquish the neoliberal role that dance often assumes as ambassador of the humanistic, the good, and the harmless, when we instead lend our bodies to pursuing violences uncoupled from cycles of harm. Cares uncoupled from carefulness. Dance that ignores bodies it doesn't like or find moral won't make those bodies go away. Dance existing in the bubble of worlds it wishes to live in, without calling in the choreographies that make such worlds so unattainable, won't conjure those worlds into being. But dance that recognizes its own history as both littered with and intrinsic to genealogies of the detestable, might have a chance to restage the past, reoccupy it, sweat the past out.

Thanks to
Anna, Annie-B, Carina, Elaine,
Frania, Karthik, Kennis, Kim, Maria,
Mango, Tamir, Tommy, V., & Varinia